CONDITIONING

Prentice-Hall Sport Series

Perry Johnson
Donald Stolberg

CONDITIONING

Prentice-Hall, Inc., Englewood Cliffs, New Jersey

QP
301
J58

C-13-167254-1
P-13-167247-9

Library of Congress Catalog Card Number 72-149308

Printed in the United States of America

Current Printing (last digit):

12 11 10 9 8 7 6 5 4 3 2 1

PRENTICE-HALL INTERNATIONAL, INC., London
PRENTICE-HALL OF AUSTRALIA, PTY. LTD., Sydney
PRENTICE-HALL OF CANADA, LTD., Toronto
PRENTICE-HALL OF INDIA PRIVATE LIMITED, New Delhi
PRENTICE-HALL OF JAPAN, INC., Tokyo

CONTENTS

I
The
First
Step

3
CAUTIONS AND SAFETY PRINCIPLES 23

4
THE CHALLENGE
physical fitness improvement 26

5
THE CHALLENGE
motor ability improvement 57

II
One
Step
Further

I

The
First
Step

1

THE PARTICIPANT

The goal of this chapter is to help you:
1. Understand the "cornerstone" of a firm foundation for
training, conditioning, and physical fitness programs
2. Understand what you need personally (physiologically,
psychologically, and in motor ability) to improve physical
fitness or to benefit by some specific training program
3. Be aware of the broad range of requisites, other
than your personal qualities, for participation
in training and physical fitness programs

"Toads have the power of sucking the poison of cancer from the system." Wearing eel skin garters will prevent muscle cramps in the legs. The remedy for a swollen knee is to "kill a cat, split the body lengthwise, and apply it, while warm, to the knee, binding it thereon, and let it stay there 'til the cure is complete." These superstitions (Radford and Radford, 1949) are laughable to most of us. Yet many who would laugh at these health superstitions accept at face value equally ridiculous concepts about health and physical fitness. Some people really believe that hairy chests are a sign of strength. We know at least one person who teaches that physical fitness will prevent cancer. We are not suggesting that you are naive enough to believe any of these particular superstitions. These are obviously extreme examples; but they do serve to introduce the concept that is the cornerstone of a sound foundation for understanding training (a program for improving skilled performance), conditioning (a program for increasing the physiological capacity of one or more systems of the body), and physical fitness (the capacity to meet the demands of reasonably vigorous physical activity). That cornerstone is knowledge, not superstition or fad, about what these things can do for you and, of equal importance, what they cannot do for you.

WHAT YOU NEED

What qualities do you need to be able to benefit from a training or conditioning program? You need first of all to have a purpose firmly in mind; and second, to know what benefits you can expect and what the limits are on your chances for success. You may wish to raise your general physical fitness level to improve health or well-being, or to prepare for possible emergency situations in which greater physical fitness would be desirable. On the other hand, you may wish to develop specific kinds of physical fitness (let us say strength) or motor ability (for example, speed), in order to accomplish some specific task or to improve your ability to participate in a specific sport. It is essential to keep in mind that there are *as many different training and conditioning programs as there are people who intelligently and knowledgeably use them.*

Assuming that you have identified clearly the purpose or purposes for which you intend to undertake the program, you need to face realistically at least two important questions: (1) Do I have the capacity to improve the qualities I wish to improve? (2) What are the limitations imposed by my environment, time, and so on?

Physiological Requirements

If your desire is simply to improve your level of general physical fitness, you need only have a minimal level of organic health. It is obvious, and important, that some specific organic defect may impose limitations upon the kind and amount of physical fitness you may attain. But unless you have some general disorder which makes any kind of physical effort absolutely forbidden, you can always improve your general physical fitness. Logic and common sense and, if necessary, a visit to your physician will help you balance your training or conditioning goals with your physiological capacity and limitations.

For example, it may be unreasonable for a person with some heart valve damage to expect to develop his fitness level enough to become a champion miler, but he might be able to improve and strengthen the condition of his heart and circulatory system within the limits dictated by his disorder. A blind person can undertake a conditioning program to promote his general physical fitness level; his blindness simply means that his methods may require some slight modification. Keep in mind, then, that training and conditioning programs should be highly individualized.

Psychological Requirements

Here we deal with the questions of motivation and purpose, knowledge, attitude, social interaction, and so on.

The individual who wishes to improve physical fitness or motor ability must be highly motivated to do so.

Unless one has obtained and can use certain kinds of knowledge, he may very well find himself attempting an unrealistic program or, even worse, operating on the basis of ignorance or even superstition with respect to the program in the hopes that he has for improvement. It is only with certain kinds of knowledge that you can hope to embark upon a program of any kind for any purpose that will be really and uniquely yours and tailored to your needs.

Attitude, of course, also relates to motivation and purpose. It will have a direct influence upon your persistence in meeting the challenges of any program of improvement.

Social interaction is involved in your selection of not only the means by which you intend to meet your objectives but also the very objectives themselves. For example, social needs may very well dictate improvement of physical fitness if you feel that being physically fit will make you more socially acceptable. Success in a specific sport may seem essential to social status. On the other hand, many persons may have no social reasons for improving physical fitness or motor ability. In any case, one's social needs play an important role in determining goals and the methods of attaining them. Our culture certainly affects our attitude toward health and fitness, sports participation and success therein, and so on. So you might choose to improve your physical fitness *only* if you can do so while competing with other persons, even to the extent that you would rather *not* be physically fit than have to exercise regularly by yourself in some noncompetitive or nonsocial setting. In short, the social interaction factor may be of extreme importance to some but of no importance to others.

Motor Capacity

Your degree of general motor capacity, that is, the extent to which your motor abilities can be developed, is relatively unimportant if you wish to improve general physical fitness or certain general motor abilities. On the other hand, if you wish to improve certain general motor abilities for the purpose of excelling in some sport, you should assess realistically your motor capacity and motor educability before setting goals for improvement.

Contraindications

Common sense will suffice, in most cases, to determine what disorders might preclude your participation in a given kind of training or conditioning program. It is equally important to stress that disorder or disease does not automatically preclude participation in all physical fitness improvement programs.

FACILITIES, EQUIPMENT, AND OTHER PARTICIPANTS

When you embark upon any kind of training or conditioning program, you will need some place to work, you may need some special kinds of equipment, and you may need other participants. The nature of the program determines these needs which may vary from no special facilities to highly specialized facilities, such as a swimming pool, handball court, or tennis court; from no special equipment other than exercise clothing to very specialized equipment, such as barbells and weights, or bicycles or stationary cycles; from none to many other participants, such as an opponent, a partner and two opponents, teammates and an opposing team, or a group to make otherwise unexciting and noncompetitive exercise such as jogging more enjoyable.

It is important to keep in mind that when you are preparing for a lifetime of activity which will promote or improve some quality or qualities in which you are interested, these factors—facilities, equipment, and other participants —are extremely important and can play a limiting role in the future if special needs or a sufficient number of other participants are not available.

AS YOU BEGIN YOUR PROGRAM OF TRAINING OR CONDITIONING, YOU SHOULD KEEP IN MIND THAT:

Knowledge is essential for the individual to plan sound personal fitness or training programs.

Before embarking on a program of any kind, you must have a firm purpose.

You must know what you can expect from a program, based upon knowledge of self and knowledge about the principles of training and conditioning.

Very few persons are completely unable to benefit from some form of conditioning for general fitness.

Physiological, psychological, and motor capacity factors influence individual potential for success in certain improvement endeavors, but these factors never completely prevent anyone from some form of realistic and meaningful achievement.

"Extrapersonal" needs (facilities, equipment, and other participants) vary greatly and depend upon the activity involved. There are ways to improve all aspects of fitness and motor ability without special facilities, equipment, or other persons.

2

CONCEPTS, PRINCIPLES AND DEFINITIONS

The purpose of this chapter is to help you:
1. *Understand the systems of the body and how they contribute to exercise*
2. *Become familiar with the most basic terms commonly associated with physical fitness and training programs*
3. *Understand the fundamental principles of conditioning and training*

IMPORTANT TERMS

Exercise

As used in this text, the word "exercise" refers to conscious and purposeful physical activity, usually of sufficient intensity to increase to some degree respiratory and circulatory functions. It refers only to the actual movement process at the time it occurs and should not be confused with the terms "conditioning" or "training."

Conditioning

Conditioning refers to the process by which one attempts to improve a given physiological function, which may or may not be for the purpose of bettering a skilled performance. Thus one could speak of conditioning the heart and circulatory system, conditioning the respiratory system, or conditioning certain muscle groups of the body. (It is not to be confused with the term conditioning as it is used in psychology.) Conditioning, as we use it in this text, refers to general physiological improvement of the systems of the body and not to any process whereby one attempts to improve observable and measurable motor skills. Conditioning is the process by which physical fitness qualities are improved.

Training

Training refers more to a process directed at the improvement of *performance* than does the more general term conditioning. For example, you might *train* to improve your high jumping ability but you would adopt a *conditioning* program to maintain the quality of your muscles so that you could maintain your ability to jump repeatedly in competition without fatigue. You might go into training to improve your shot put ability, but you might include as part of your program some conditioning exercises of a more general nature. In other words, one trains for the kinds of skilled performance that are measured externally, and conditions for improving the physiological capacity of a system or systems of the body. Training is the process by which motor performance is improved. It may include conditioning of one kind or another as an adjunct to improvement of performance via improvement of the contributing systems.

Physical Fitness

As defined in this text book, physical fitness is the capacity to carry out reasonably vigorous physical activities and includes qualities important to the individual's health and well-being, in general, as opposed to those that relate to performance of specific motor skills. There are only four—perhaps five—qualities basic to physical fitness. Physical fitness is attained via the process of conditioning.

Circulo-respiratory fitness (general work capacity). Circulo-respiratory fitness may also be identified as circulo-respiratory endurance or as work capacity. CR fitness is the quality that enables one to endure in reasonably vigorous physical activity for extended periods of time. Generally speaking, CR fitness is involved in activities that require the use of much of the body's large musculature (for example, running, swimming, or cycling), because these activities force the heart and circulatory system and the respiratory system to operate at a much higher level of efficiency than usual. These activities are those that must be terminated when one's circulatory and respiratory systems can no longer meet the demands of the activity, rather than because of local fatigue of a given muscle group (in other words, when labored breathing and a "pounding heart" lead to cessation rather than inability of a localized muscle group).

Muscular endurance. Muscular endurance is the quality that enables one to persist in localized muscle group activities for extended periods of time. Think of the typical tests that involve primarily local muscle groups, such as pull-ups and push-ups; these tests are usually terminated because the local muscle groups are unable to respond further, not because of inadequate performance of the circulo-respiratory system in general which is usually characterized by labored breathing and a noticeably pounding heart.

Strength. A great deal of confusion has surrounded the use of the term "strength." Quite often it has been erroneously associated with such activities as pull-ups and push-ups. We have just indicated that these activities depend upon the quality of muscular endurance. Strength may be properly defined as maximal force exerted one time. *Isometric* strength is the maximal amount of force one can exert against a fixed resistance during one all-out application. *Isotonic* (dynamic) strength is properly defined as the amount of resistance one can overcome during one application of force through the full range of motion of the particular joint or joints of the body involved (an arm curl with barbell, for example). Strength is, of course, specific to a given muscle or muscle group and is dependent upon the nature of the resistance, that is, whether it is fixed or movable.

We may further clarify the difference between strength and muscular endurance by using an analogy. The strength of a wooden beam expected to support the weight of some structure is measured by its ability to support a given amount of weight and not by the length of time it will be able to support that weight. One would expect, of course, that strength and muscular endurance would be related, and it is obvious that a muscle group capable of exerting a maximum of 100 pounds of force through the full range of motion would be capable of repeatedly moving a 20-pound weight through the full range of motion (at a given rate) more times than would a muscle group capable of exerting a maximum of 30 pounds of force through the full range of motion.

Flexibility. Flexibility is defined as the functional capacity of a joint to move through a normal range of motion. It is specific to given joints and is actually more dependent upon the musculature surrounding a joint than on the actual bony structure of the joint itself (except in cases of disease or disorder of the skeletal system or its joints).

Body composition. We list this tentatively as a quality of physical fitness because at the present time there is considerable evidence that excess fat stored in the body limits health and physical fitness.

Motor Capacity

"Motor capacity," as used in this text, refers to the extent to which one can develop his motor abilities.

Motor Educability

"Motor educability" refers to one's ability to adapt to and learn new movements or activities that depend to a high degree upon motor performance.

Motor Ability

Motor ability is, as the name suggests, the ability to carry out particular motor functions. We have classified these functions as follows.

Coordination. Coordination is most likely an essential part of all the other motor ability parameters. It may be defined as the smooth flow of movement in the execution of a motor task. It involves the blending of forceful and explosive movements with accurate and less forceful movements and the sequential blending of different movements to achieve some purposeful movement.

Balance. "Balance" is the ability to maintain one's equilibrium while stationary and while moving in various ways at various speeds.

Power. Power is involved whenever the desired result requires explosive movement of the body. The vertical jump, the shot put, the baseball throw, and sprinting are all examples of power movements. A great amount of force must be applied over as short a period of time as possible to achieve the optimal result.

Agility. Agility is generally defined as the ability to change direction quickly and effectively while moving as nearly as possible at full speed.

Speed. Speed is defined as the ability to move the entire body rapidly from one place to another.

Movement time. Movement time differs from speed in that it involves the movement of a *part* of the body from one point to another. For example, one might measure the movement time involved in the specific pattern of the arm and shoulder movement during the shot put.

Reaction time. Reaction time is the length of time required to initiate a response to a specific stimulus. When movement time is added to reaction time, we have what is commonly called response time.

THE SYSTEMS OF THE BODY AND HOW THEY CONTRIBUTE
TO EXERCISE

To understand the principles of training and conditioning, it is helpful to possess at least some fundamental knowledge about each system of the body and how it contributes to exercise.

The Nervous System

The task of communication between various segments of the body and the integration of its many complex activities are responsibilities shared by the nervous system with the endocrine system. The autonomic system (controlling the heart, intestines, urogenital tract, blood vessels, endocrine glands, and so on) is one division of the nervous system and the somatic system (controlling the sensory impulses and motor responses of the skeletal musculature) the other. The autonomic system is frequently called the "involuntary" nervous system, because it is not under the conscious control of the individual. The somatic system is concerned with activation of skeletal muscle, either as the result of a conscious wish or entirely from reflex, though reflexes involving the somatic system can be consciously overridden.

The nervous system is involved not only in initiating, coordinating, and directing activity, but also is largely responsible for producing the necessary adjustment in body functions to make the exercise possible. Some of these functions and the portions of the nervous system responsible for them are listed below:

Cerebrum—sensations, voluntary movements, memory of skills, judgment, all conscious functions.

Thalamus—complex reflex movements, perception of sensations.

Hypothalamus—coordination of autonomic functions; control of body temperature by sweating, constriction of dilation of blood vessels, shivering, and so on.

Cerebellum—coordination of skilled movements, maintenance of equilibrium through action on skeletal muscles, necessary for smooth and effective movements.

Medulla Oblongata—contains reflex centers that regulate heart rate, blood pressure, and respiratory rate and depth.

The Muscular System

Although we are concerned mainly with that function of the muscles which produces body movement, it should also be mentioned that muscles are responsible for producing most of the body heat as well as for maintaining upright posture. There are three distinct kinds of muscle tissue: (1) skeletal or striated muscle, (2) cardiac or heart muscle, and (3) smooth muscle, such as is found in blood vessels and the intestines. This discussion is limited to a consideration of skeletal muscle. Any adequate discussion of skeletal muscle function must take into account the interdependent nature of the muscular system, the nervous system, and the skeletal system. The muscular and nervous systems are needed to cause the muscles to contract at the proper time and in the appropriate sequence, and the skeletal system provides the system of levers through which the muscles are able to accomplish work.

The characteristic that distinguishes muscle from all other tissue is its ability to contract. In fact, only by shortening do muscles perform work. They can perform "negative" work, such as that involved in lowering oneself from a high bar, by gradually lengthening the shortened muscle (known as eccentric contraction). The many muscles of the body are made up of thousands of tiny contractile fibers grouped together into bundles. These bundles in turn are grouped together into muscles of many different shapes and sizes. The force with which a given muscle contracts depends upon the number of individual fibers that are actually stimulated at once and the frequency with which they are stimulated. These factors enable us to perform smoothly such diverse actions as playing a piano, or lifting it.

Each muscle fiber is supplied (innervated) by a single motor nerve fiber (neuron). Branches of the same neuron may innervate several separate muscle fibers. This arrangement of a single motor neuron together with all of the muscle fibers that it innervates is called a motor unit. Whenever such a motor neuron is activated, it causes *all* of its individual muscle fibers to contract. Thus, muscles involved in very delicate adjustments (such as those controlling eye movements) would have motor units made up of fewer muscle fibers per nerve fiber than muscles that are generally concerned with gross activity (such as jumping).

The Circulatory and Respiratory Systems

The primary function of the circulatory system may be stated in one simple word—transport. This system transports essentials, like glucose and oxygen, to the cells and waste materials, like carbon dioxide, from the cells. The respiratory system exists for the primary purpose of supplying oxygen to the cells and removing carbon dioxide from them. But for this to take place the circulatory system must aid the respiratory system by transporting the oxygen and carbon dioxide between the lungs and cells. There are four basic aspects of total respiration: lung ventilation (breathing); external respiration (exchange of O_2 and CO_2 between the air-sacs of the lungs and the blood); internal respiration (exchange of O_2 and CO_2 at the cell membrane); true respiration (the actual oxidative process within the cell walls).

The most important functional parts of the circulatory system are the heart, the blood, and the vascular bed. The heart is composed of specialized tissue known as cardiac muscle and is innately rhythmic. It has its own rich blood supply (coronary arteries) and needs nutrients and oxygen in order to function just as skeletal or smooth muscles do. Consisting of four chambers and a series of valves, it serves as the pump to circulate and recirculate blood throughout the closed vascular system.

The vascular bed consists of the large arteries, small arteries, arterioles, capillaries, venules, small veins, and large veins. The arterioles contain smooth muscle fibers in their walls (under the control of the autonomic nervous system) and thus can constrict or dilate. This change in diameter serves to alter general systemic blood pressure and blood flow to particular areas of the body, which is very important in exercise. Very slight changes in the arteriolar diameter cause dramatic changes in blood flow.

As one would expect, the circulatory system is called upon to increase its transport of essentials to the cells and waste products from the cells during muscular exertion. This increase, of course, is directly related to the intensity and duration of exertion. Cessation of activities involving much of the body's musculature in long term, rhythmic movement (for example, jogging and distance swimming) is partly determined by the capacity of this system to meet the oxygen needs of the tissues. Total blood flow, or cardiac output, is increased in even the mildest activity. It may increase to as much as 35 liters per minute in a highly conditioned male, or as much as a seven-fold increase over resting blood flow. This increase is the result of increases in both heart rate and stroke volume though some evidence indicates that exercise causes the stroke volume of sedentary individuals to increase very little, and that the increase in cardiac output is due almost entirely to an increased heart rate.

Whatever the mechanism, the increased output speeds delivery of essentials to and waste materials from the working muscles. Because of increased blood flow to muscles and constriction of arterioles in the non-involved areas of the body, such as the stomach and the skin, systolic blood pressure rises during exertion. This increased working pressure, along with a concurrent arteriolar dilatation in the muscles, means increased blood flow through the working muscles. Flow to the brain remains relatively constant, and cardiac blood flow increases. Thus the blood is not only circulated faster, but it is circulated to the areas where it is most needed during exertion. When heat dissipation becomes inadequate, the thermoregulatory center, via the autonomic nervous system, causes arteriolar dilatation in the skin. This allows the flowing blood to act as a radiator system and increases heat loss, because the blood is so close to the surface of the skin. It is possible that the spleen ejects some of its reserve red blood cells into circulation during exercise to increase the capacity for carrying oxygen and carbon dioxide.

During even the mildest exertion the cells increase their demand for oxygen. In response to this demand, the entire respiratory system steps up its activity. The actual degree of increase in respiratory functions naturally depends upon the intensity and duration of the exertion. Both the depth (tidal volume) and rate of breathing increase: the ventilation rate may increase from a resting level of 6-10 liters per minute to as high as 120-150 liters per minute in a trained person.

As a result of these changes, oxygen utilization may increase to as high as 4000-6000 milliliters per minute from a resting value of 200-350 milliliters per minute. If oxygen utilization does not equal the oxygen requirement, one can still continue activity until he reaches his maximal oxygen debt tolerance. This ability of the muscles to function anaerobically (without oxygen) allows us to perform tasks we otherwise could not perform. Generally speaking, sprints are oxygen debt-producing or anaerobic events, whereas distance events are aerobic or "steady state" events. (When oxygen utilization equals the oxygen requirement, then oxygen utilization and heart rate level off and one can continue the effort for a longer period of time. This leveling off is referred to as a "steady state" and can be observed only in submaximal work tasks, not in all-out exertion).

The Digestive System

The function of the digestive system is simply to prepare food for the processes of absorption and metabolism. Generally speaking, the digestive system has little if any function during the actual exercise period. There may be exceptions in the case of very long marathon runs or distance swimming, during which food may be ingested in order to supply needed energy. Usually, however, all the energy has already been supplied and stored in some form in the body. Because the absorption of food is a rather slow process, eating immediately before or during a contest would usually be of little if any benefit. Of course, it is important that proper nutritional practices be followed if sufficient energy stores are to be available to sustain vigorous activity. The energy for muscle contraction is derived from the combination of oxygen with energy-rich compounds, which have been stored in the muscles and elsewhere. Limitations on performance are set by the extent of availability of oxygen and the food-derived energy sources (glucose, fats, proteins) as well as by the accumulation of the waste products of metabolism, such as CO_2 and lactic acid.

The Endocrine System

The ductless glands of the endocrine system secrete hormones that aid in controlling many functions of the other systems of the body. Many are essential for life and for the increased function of the systems during exercise.

The pituitary gland is known as the master gland because it controls or works reciprocally with most of the other endocrine glands. The thyroid gland secretes the hormone thyroxin which controls the metabolic rate of the body's cells but has no short range effect during exercise *per se*. The Islets of Langerhans, located in the pancreas, secrete insulin which is essential for transporting glucose across the cell membranes. The adrenal glands are particularly active during exercise. The outer portion of these tiny glands secretes epinephrine, commonly called adrenalin, which supports the sympathetic nervous system in increasing systemic blood pressure, increases blood glucose, and generally prepares the systems in many ways for "flight or fight." The inner or cortical portion of the adrenals secretes three classes of hormones, two of which are particularly important in exercise. The mineralocorticoids assist in controlling body water and electrolyte balance, and the glucocorticoids are essential to the increased demands for energy metabolism.

The Skin

Although not ordinarily thought of as a system in the same sense as the circulatory system or the nervous system, the highly specialized cells that form the skin do make up an extremely important structure. The functions of the skin include such diverse elements as protection, excretion, maintenance of fluid and electrolyte balance; the latter two are of special importance in exercise.

Sensation is, of course, essential to human survival in an environment that contains many harmful and dangerous elements. Sensitivity to pain, for example, tends to cause the organism to avoid situations that might cause injury. Tactile sensation (sense of touch) aids in the skillful manipulation of objects, including those used in sports and games.

The interaction of the human body and its environment with respect to temperature is one which deserves special consideration. The sense organs that respond to heat or cold supply essential information to help the body avoid serious malfunction owing to excessive loss of heat or to excessive heat retention. In a cold environment the blood vessels near the surface of the skin become constricted so that the blood does not lose heat to the cold surroundings. In exercise, the capillaries near the surface become filled with blood and a great deal of heat is lost to the atmosphere by radiation from the surface of the body. When external temperature is high, however, there may be too little difference between body temperature and environmental temperature for heat to be lost by radiation. In such cases evaporation becomes the chief means by which heat can be dissipated. The sweat glands secrete a watery fluid which, in evaporating from the surface of the skin, causes an effective reduction of skin temperature. Thus, blood that absorbs heat from active muscles can be shunted to the vessels of the skin where the excessive heat can be lost through radiation and evaporation. Indeed, the ability of the body to dissipate excess heat in this manner is an important limiting factor in exercise under certain conditions. Failure to carry off excessive heat results in heat exhaustion and sometimes even death. Thus, it is easy to see that when both environmental temperature and humidity are high, the two major means of heat dissipation are seriously restricted. Under such circumstances one is unable to engage in as much vigorous physical activity as usual.

The Skeletal System

In everyday activity the skeletal system has five important functions.

1. It provides protection for vital organs of the body: for example, the skull protects the brain.

2. It supports the body just as girders support buildings.

3. It affords a means of movement. Muscles attached to bones contract, and these bones, with their joints, act as levers to create movement.

4. Bones serve as a storage depot for calcium needed by other body systems.

5. The red bone marrow manufactures blood cells, usually all the red cells in the adult and most types of white blood cells as well as the blood platelets.

The increased demands upon the circulatory system in protracted exercise or training create the need for more red cells in order to increase the oxygen carrying capacity of the blood. In addition, the added wear and tear (friction, pressure, and so forth) on the cells that accompanies training shortens their life span, further increasing the need for new cells. The bone marrow of the long and flat bones of the body responds to this need.

The essential role of the skeleton as a system of levers making exercise possible is obvious. Not quite so obvious is the fact that most of these levers are of the third class (force located between fulcrum and resistance) thus making the body better adapted for speed than force.

The Liver

The liver is not generally considered to be a system, but it will be discussed briefly because of its importance in exercise. It is difficult to present a simple description of its purpose, as some 500 functions are attributed to the liver. These functions may be categorized as follows:

1. Storage of materials (for example, glycogen, fat).

2. Manufacture and conversion of materials (for example, certain anti-bodies, bile, glycogen, fat, certain vitamins).

3. Detoxification (removal of certain impurities from blood).

4. Creation of body heat (creates about 20 percent of total body heat).

5. Some blood storage in its sinuses.

6. Aiding of certain endocrine glands.

The liver contributes to exercise indirectly in many ways, but it affects exercise directly in three basic ways.

1. Adequate glucose levels in the blood and tissues during exercise are maintained to a large extent by liver glycogenolysis and gluconeogenesis; therefore work capacity is greater.

2. Exercise can continue anaerobically for a limited period of time. The ability of the liver to convert lactic acid to glycogen or glucose, in the presence of oxygen, retards the accumulation of an oxygen debt and thus contributes to steady state performance, thereby increasing work capacity.

3. By converting lactic acid, the liver plays a role in maintaining blood pH within normal limits. This conversion of lactic acid also increases the carbon dioxide-carrying capacity of the blood because the removing of lactic acid frees one of the carbon dioxide-carrying media.

Excretory System

The excretory system, composed of the kidneys, skin, respiratory tract, and digestive tract, is concerned with removal of waste products. The kidneys filter the blood (about one-quarter of the blood volume is filtered per minute) and excrete excess materials as well as waste products such as urea, uric acid and creatinine. In addition to water, some carbon dioxide is eliminated through the skin, although most of it is blown off by the lungs. Some water vapor is also lost in ventilation. The waste products eliminated by the digestive tract in the form of feces are the unabsorbed products of digestion.

Blood volume is affected to a large extent by the kidneys' excretion of water. During exercise, blood flow to the kidneys is reduced and therefore less blood is filtered. As a result, less urine is formed and blood volume is reduced less severely. It is probable that the antidiuretic hormone of the posterior pituitary, which increases renal water reabsorption, comes into play to further conserve plasma. These renal functions help to maintain systemic blood pressure and also provide additional water for heat dissipation through sweating. It is obvious that increased ventilation results from exercise. One of the most powerful stimuli for this increase is excess CO_2 in the blood. By increasing CO_2 removal, the respiratory system plays a very important role in maintenance of a near-normal blood pH value during exercise.

FUNDAMENTAL PRINCIPLES OF TRAINING AND CONDITIONING

You are probably well aware of requirements for improvement in physical fitness even though you may not be able to articulate them. Experimentation has supported observation and intuitive beliefs concerning what it takes to cause improvement. These principles are commonly referred to as the principles of demand (overload) and specificity.

"Demand" expresses the principle that great demands must be placed on a system if significant changes are to occur. For example, how can the heart be strengthened if no demand is ever placed upon it other than that of a very inactive and sedentary existence? Why would a muscle group be expected to increase in strength if it is never asked to exert force against any resistance greater than 25 percent of what it is already capable of exerting? In other words, the physiological response of the systems of the body occurs because of a particular *need* for that response.

It is important to keep in mind that this principle apparently holds true for any kind of improvement in conditioning or training. That is to say, even where an increase in musculature is not involved, a demand must be *repeatedly* placed upon the system or systems involved if improvement is to occur. Improvement in a particular kind of coordination, for example, juggling three balls at once or executing a swan dive, involves placing the demand for that coordinated act upon the neuromuscular system. If this demand is not placed upon the system, no improvement will occur. The systems of the body respond in many unseen ways to the demands placed upon them (for example, increased stroke volume of the heart, more consistent patterns of muscle fiber contraction for a given skill, and so on).

The demand principle is often expressed in another way. We speak of the *law of use and disuse* which simply means that an organ or system that is used maintains or improves its capacity to function, whereas an organ that is not used tends to lose its functional capacity. This law is best exemplified by the changes that can occur in the musculature of the body. Hypertrophy (increased muscle size) can occur as a result of great demands placed upon a muscle group. A trip to "muscle beach" or to the nearest weight lifting club will provide dramatic examples of how extensive muscle hypertrophy can be. The exact opposite, atrophy (wasting of the muscle), can occur as a result of complete immobility, and is often seen as the result of prolonged immobilization of a limb which has been broken and placed for some period of time in a cast.

Simply stated, "specificity" of training and conditioning means that "you get what you work for." An extreme example will serve to illustrate this principle. One would not expect to become a championship swimmer if his training program were composed only of weight lifting and running. Neither would one expect to become a championship miler by spending two hours a day in the swimming pool. There are, of course, less obvious examples of disregard for this very important principle. A high school student progressed from 10 to 75 push-ups per day over a period of six weeks and then complained that he had not increased the size or "definition" of his biceps! Athletes have been known to run cross-country in order to prepare for the basketball season only to be perplexed by the fact that they still developed blisters and sore muscles when they began basketball practice.

Ignorance of the principle of specificity can easily lead to frustration. On the other hand, obedience to this principle should in most cases provide you with the soundest training and conditioning program. Keep in mind that nothing replaces the activity itself if you wish to improve it and that the second best activity is one that simulates as nearly as possible the activity or movement you wish to improve. Thus, for example, we have found it more profitable to use overload jumping to improve one's vertical jumping ability than to use the more traditional squats or semisquats and the rise-on-toes. Certainly the latter two exercises involve the same muscles that we use in jumping. Yet they do not do so at the same rate of muscle contraction that we employ in actually jumping vertically. This is not to say that there is no benefit to be derived from nonspecific kinds of physical fitness conditioning. But if you wish to improve a capacity or a specific skill, the best approach is to practice that activity.

Other Principles

Most other training and conditioning principles fall into one of two categories: (1) general principles of learning, and (2) specific principles relating to each given activity or skill. General learning principles will be dealt with in Part II of this text and specific principles will be dealt with as we discuss each activity or exercise.

One principle, not as firmly established as the two basic principles of demand and specificity, bears mentioning. Most persons who have been involved in any kind of training, conditioning, or learning process have at some time encountered what is often called a "plateau" or a "sticking point." (Some practitioners and scientists have used the term *retrogression*.) Retrogression simply means that we can often expect a period of leveling off or even falling off in performance after some improvement has taken place. Some people have tried to relate this phenomenon to what is commonly known as "staleness." The exact mechanism or cause for such retrogression has not been unequivocally established but it happens often enough to warrant comment. Whether it is primarily physiological or psychological is immaterial at this point. But it is important that you be prepared for it so that you will not become discouraged. Although there is no certain cure, there are several successful approaches, all of which, in effect, interrupt the training or conditioning program for a day or two. For example, you may practice a diversionary activity for a day or two. Such an interruption often results in improved success or an improved performance upon return to the routine.

Basic Mechanical Principles

Some basic mechanical principles are important to success in a given activity or skill and some are essential for safety. Although these are often very general in nature, we feel it best to discuss most of them in connection with the specific activities. However, because the mechanical principles of applying force are important for safety as well as achievement of mechanical advantage in all kinds of activities, they are summarized here (Massey et. al., 1959).

1. *Leverage.* The length of the lever arm influences the effective force that can be applied. For example, a weight held with the arms extended straight out to the side requires more force than a weight directly supported over the flexed elbows.

2. *Angle of Pull.* The angle at which a force acts upon a limb or lever determines the force that rotates a limb about its joint and the force that stabilizes a joint. The maximum force of pull, in terms of rotation, occurs at $90°$. A muscle exerts its maximum rotatory pull on a bone at the point at which it pulls at a nearly vertical angle with the bone. In other words, the greatest force or resistance to force can usually be applied when a joint is at approximately a $90°$ angle.

3. *Center of Gravity.* In lifting, in order to maintain body balance, the center of gravity must always be kept within the area that can be supported by the base of support. For instance, the center of gravity of a heavy barbell must be carefully selected in order to control the weight during critical parts of the lift.

Particularly from a safety standpoint, it is important to know that the leg muscles, not the back muscles, are the strongest in the body. Therefore, when lifting a heavy weight, you should squat, with the back relatively erect, and lift the weight by straightening (extending) the knees and hip joint.

YOU SHOULD NOW UNDERSTAND THAT:

Exercise, conditioning, training, physical fitness, and motor ability are not interchangeable terms.

Each of the body's systems, including the skin and the liver, contribute in some essential way to the adaptation to exercise. An understanding of these functions can aid you in planning for fitness or motor ability improvement.

There are two common denominators for all training and conditioning methods: demand and specificity.

Retrogression often occurs in fitness or motor ability improvement programs and should not be viewed with alarm or discouragement.

3

CAUTIONS AND SAFETY
PRINCIPLES

The purpose of this chapter is to help you become aware of:
1. General safety principles
2. Precautionary measures associated
with training and conditioning

You should never engage in physical activity unless you are reasonably certain that you are physically prepared to do so. Whether or not you are prepared depends on several factors: age, current fitness level, general health, and particular activity involved. For example, there is practically no health risk to a fifteen-year-old, in good general health, if he participates in a 100-yard dash at a family picnic, even if he is in a very low state of physical fitness. On the other hand, a 45-year-old man who is in good general health but at a very low level of general physical fitness would be taking a considerably greater health risk. Another 45-year-old, who has maintained an excellent state of physical fitness all his life, could participate in the dash with little more health risk than the fifteen-year-old. This same kind of common sense applies to any kind of activity. It applies to the initiation of long-range programs as well as to one-shot participation.

The precautionary principle might be stated in this manner: the older you are, the lower your general physical fitness level, the poorer your general state of health, and the more vigorous the activity, then the greater your moderation in physical activity should be.

An ancillary principle would be: the older you are, the poorer your fitness state, the poorer your general health status, and the more vigorous the proposed activity program, the more important it becomes for you to have a thorough physical examination before beginning the program. As an example, an eighteen-year-old who is in good health and who had an annual physical six months ago could proceed without undue concern to participate in a jogging program; a man fifty years of age, even having had a general physical examination six months ago, should probably have a more specific physical examination before plunging into such a vigorous fitness program.

The question of warm-up is usually raised in connection with cautions and safety principles, and although there is some experimental evidence that warm-up is of questionable value, it still seems sensible for reducing the chance of muscle injury resulting from sudden and forceful overloaded movements. At any rate it is not likely to have any harmful effects as a part of a fitness program.

We will suggest specific precautions and safety principles in connection with certain activities and programs. There are, however, a few more principles that deserve your attention in a more general context.

1. As a general rule, most muscle injuries sustained during physical activity, either impact-type injuries or muscle or tendon pulls, should be treated by the application of ice or cold water, elastic pressure wrap, elevation, and rest, not by the application of heat.

2. Following unconsciousness or semiconsciousness resulting from a blow or even from overexhaustion, it is wise to discontinue the activity. Although unconsciousness and semiconsciousness do not always indicate damage to brain tissues, the possibility of damage is real and should not be treated lightly.

3. Pay particular attention to your body's need for water as expressed by thirst, and resist the temptation to give in to the myth that wearing heavy sweat clothing and rubber suits will lead to permanent weight loss if worn while exercising. The *very* small possible weight reduction value is more than counterbalanced by the very real threat of dehydration, heat stroke, and even death.

4. After the age of thirty, and particularly if you are in poor physical condition, it is advisable not to participate in vigorous exercise alone.

IN YOUR CONDITIONING ENDEAVORS, ALWAYS BE CAREFUL TO:

Choose your activities to fit your present physical condition.

Be alert for bodily cues that you are placing too much strain on your body or any of its systems.

4

THE CHALLENGE
physical fitness improvement

The purpose of this chapter is to help you:
1. *Learn how to test for the five*
   physical fitness qualities
2. *Understand the basic principles*
   of physical fitness improvement
3. *Become familiar with the general methods and examples*
   of basic programs designed to improve physical fitness
4. *Become aware of more specific programs*
   for improving physical fitness

CIRCULO-RESPIRATORY FITNESS

Tests

There are several good laboratory tests of lung capacity, breathing capacity, and circulo-respiratory adaptation to physical work. Among these are tests of vital capacity (which measures the total capacity of the lungs), maximal breathing capacity (which measures the amount of air you can move into and out of the lungs per minute), the PWC170 test (Wahlund, 1948) (which determines the length of time it takes you to reach the heart rate of 170 beats per minute through a standard progressive exercise, usually on a stationary bicycle), the maximal oxygen utilization test (which determines the greatest amount of oxygen your body is capable of using during all-out work), and the modifications of what is known as a step test.

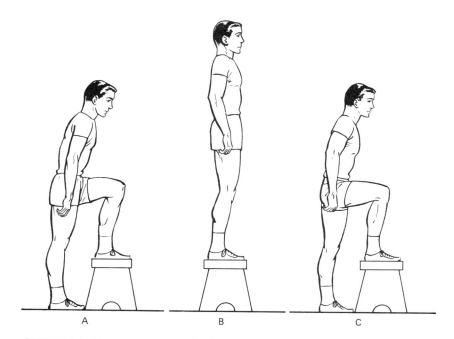

A   B   C

FIGURE 4-1. Step test to measure circulo-respiratory fitness

Of these tests, the only one practical in the nonlaboratory setting is the last. Step tests involve alternate stepping up and down at a given rate or cadence (Fig. 4-1) using a bench, chair, or stool ranging in height from 8'' to 20''. The stepping goes on for a given length of time and then the post-exercise heart rate is recorded to estimate one's adaptation to the standard work load. Variations of the step test are presented for your use (tables 4-1—4-3), but so long as you keep the general principles in mind, any adaptation, so long as it places sufficient demand on the circulo-respiratory system, will probably be adequate. The general principles for using the step test are as follows:

1. Always take the test at approximately the same time of day, especially if you wish to compare your results to determine whether improvement has taken place. (There is quite normally a diurnal variation in resting heart rate which can easily affect your results.)

2. Take the test under approximately the same conditions (time and

amount of last meal, prior physical activity, freedom from infection, amount of sleep, and so on).

3. Always use a bench of the same height.

4. Always step at the same rate (using a metronome or a record with a beat of about thirty counts per minute, if you wish).

5. Standardize the length of the test.

6. Count the heart rate by placing the fingers at the radial pulse (wrist) or carotid pulse (just to the right or left of the Adam's apple; do not press too hard here since the pressure can alter the heart rate).

7. Especially when unfit, do not be ashamed of stopping before reaching your projected time limit. This may simply be an indication of your lack of CR fitness, and you can record the time at which you were forced to stop. You can continue to work toward the state of CR fitness that will eventually allow you to complete the test.

8. Because many factors can affect the recovery heart rate, do not be discouraged if, after some time spent in a conditioning program, great improvement in heart rate response does not occur. Simply repeat the test under the conditions outlined above.

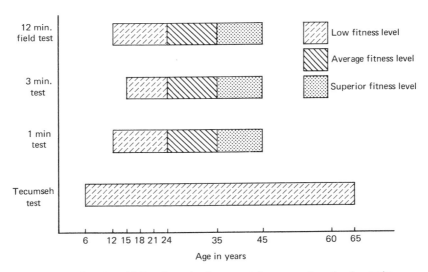

FIGURE 4-2. Rough guideline for selecting a test for measuring circulo-respiratory fitness

In addition to the three variations of the step test, we have included Cooper's Twelve-Minute Field Test (Cooper, 1968). Figure 4-2 shows you how to select the most appropriate test, depending upon your age, sex, and estimated current fitness level.

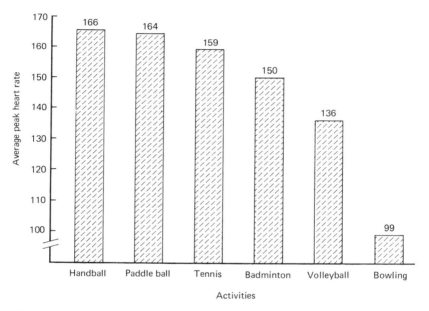

FIGURE 4-3. Peak heart rates in college males during various activities (based on Kozar and Hunsicker, 1963)

General Principles for Improvement

1. Considerable demand must be placed upon the circulo-respiratory system if improvement in its capacity is to occur. An excellent index of this demand is the exercising (see Fig. 4-3) and post-exercise heart rate. Unless exercise is of considerable duration, one cannot expect measurable gains in circulo-respiratory capacity. A heart rate of at least 140-150 beats per minute should be achieved for at least eight to ten minutes several times per week (Sharkey and Holloman, 1962). The demand necessary to produce gains, of course, depends upon the individual, his current level of circulo-respiratory fitness, and other factors.

TABLE 4-1.
Tecumseh Submaximal Exercise Test[a]:
for ages 10-69 (unless in poor health); 8" bench; 24 steps per minute, for 3 minutes

	PULSE COUNT	SCORING
Method A	Time 10 heart beats 1 minute after exercise	600/X, where X = time (to nearest tenth of a second) for 10 heart beats
Method B	Count heart beats for 15 seconds beginning 1 minute after exercise	Multiply count by 4

Norms (Percentile)	HEARTBEATS, MEN	HEARTBEATS, WOMEN
95th (excellent)	67	75
75th (above average)	79	85
50th (average)	90	95
25th (poor)	100	110

[a]Adapted from H. J. Montoye, P. W. Willis III, and D. A. Cunningham, "Heart Rate Response to Submaximal Exercise: Relation to Age and Sex," *Journal of Gerontology,* 1968, *23*, 127.

TABLE 4-2.
Michael-Adams One Minute Step Test[a]:
for young adults in good physical condition, using 17" bench for one minute

Rate:
    Men: 36 steps per minute
    Women: 30 steps per minute

Pulse count:
    From 1 minute to 1 minute 15 seconds after exercise
    From 2 minutes to 2 minutes 15 seconds after exercise
    From 3 minutes to 3 minutes 15 seconds after exercise

Scoring
    Total the three counts, multiply by 4

Norm:
    Average score for men and women: 300

[a]Adapted from E. D. Michael and A. Adams, "The Use of the One-Minute Step Test to Estimate Exercise Fitness," *Ergonomics,* 1964, *7*, 211.

TABLE 4-3.
Modified Step Test:
for young adults; 17" bench; 30 steps per minute (metronome = 120); 3 minutes for men, 2 minutes for women

	PULSE COUNT	SCORING
	From 1 minute to 1 minute and 30 seconds after exercise	Multiply count by 2
Norms:	MEN	WOMEN
Excellent	Below 100	Below 110
Above average	100-110	110-120
Average	111-124	121-134
Poor	Above 125	Above 135

2. Total musculature. The greater the proportion of total body musculature involved in the activity, the greater the demand placed on the CR system. Thus running, for example, is a better CR activity than pull-ups or push-ups since the leg muscles are considerably larger than arm and shoulder girdle muscles. Propelling the body forward, upward, or both without mechanical assistance is best; if movement of the arms is involved, the demand becomes even greater.

3. Intensity. For a given amount of musculature, the greater the intensity of activity, the greater will be the demand. For example, the demand is greater in sprinting than in jogging. This does not mean that the "fastest" activities are necessarily the best for promoting CR fitness. There is a point of no return, so to speak, at which intensity becomes so great that duration is reduced severely; CR fitness will then be less than if intensity were reduced and duration increased.

4. Duration. Duration can become so great, if there is a drastic reduction

TABLE 4-4.
Rating scale for 12-minute field test[a]

IF YOU COVER:	YOUR FITNESS CATEGORY IS:
1.75 miles or more	Excellent
1.50-1.74 miles	Good
1.25-1.49 miles	Fair
1.0-1.24 miles	Poor
Less than 1.0 miles	Very poor

[a]From Cooper, 1968.

in intensity, that little if any CR fitness can be achieved. To illustrate, one could walk slowly for hours without much CR benefit. A reasonable combination of intensity and duration is best.

5. Regularity. Although there is some evidence that for certain kinds of programs, two or three workouts per week may be as beneficial as four or five per week, it is obvious that regularity is essential to CR fitness improvement. Irregular physical activity cannot be expected to improve the fitness level.

6. Beginning point and rate of advance. The level of strenuousness and the rate at which that level is increased from day to day and week to week is an individual matter. A good rule of thumb is: be conservative and underestimate rather than overestimate your capacity. If you are in doubt, begin any program at the lowest level suggested. Then if you find that level far too easy, adjust upward. An older person or a particularly unfit person who starts above his level may never have the opportunity to adjust downward!

Methods and Programs for Improvement

There is seemingly an infinite number of approaches to intelligent development of CR capacity. Obviously we cannot present all of these in detail, but can recommend those programs and activities we feel are practical. We have indicated the lowest starting level and the goal toward which the normal healthy individual might work. You must develop your own pace of progression from the lowest to the highest level. However, if you wish more specific guides, refer to the recommended programs which often provide week-by-week schedules for attainment of the desired capacity.

The program or activity that you select will have to be based on at least three critical factors: (1) What do you like to do? (2) What facilities are available to you? and (3) How much time do you have to devote to the program? A fourth factor may be involved: are other persons necessary? The one factor about which you will have little knowledge at this point is that of time required. We have indicated for each activity and program the time, in minutes per day and number of times per week, required to progress from the lowest level to the optimal level of CR capacity through that activity or program (Table 4-5).

Two common denominators for all programs and activities are:

1. Approximately 10 to 15 weeks are required to move to the optimal or final level (10 for the reasonably fit person and 15 for the person who starts at the lowest level of fitness).

2. All programs should probably begin at a frequency of three days of activity per week for one or two weeks, then five days per week until the optimal level is obtained, at which time three or four days per week will be sufficient.

The activities are presented (Table 4-5) in order from those that ultimately require the greatest daily investment of time down to the ones which require the least time per day. (Only actual activity time is considered, since travel to and from a particular facility will vary.)

Specific Programs

Some programs provide specific information as to day-by-day and week-by-week progression, utilizing a specific activity as the means to improve circulo-respiratory capacity. We recommend that you examine the following programs.

1. *Jogging* (Bowerman and Harris, 1967) This is a systematized approach to jogging for fitness.

2. *Aerobics* (Cooper, 1968) This is a highly systematized approach utilizing your choice of many different activities.

3. *Adult Physical Fitness* (1963) This is the more traditional fitness program.

You should also be aware of two rather specialized concepts that can be used in CR conditioning programs. The first of these is circuit training which involves moving from station to station for various fitness exercises. (A special section is devoted to this concept; see page 66.) The second concept is interval training. Interval training is a form of progressive conditioning that involves the varying of the different factors involved in the conditioning program. The basic premise is that the work to be accomplished is divided into units. Each unit is, of course, accomplished at an intensity greater than would be possible if the activity were to be carried on for a longer period of time. It is possible to vary the following factors: (1) intensity of the activity (that is, the rate of accomplishment), (2) duration of each unit or bout of activity, (3) number of bouts, and (4) time and nature of the rest periods between bouts. It is also possible to vary the bouts so that some are more intense and of shorter duration than others during the same workout period. This leads to another possibility for variation, changing the order of the various bouts when they differ in intensity and duration. It is often the goal of interval training to increase the intensity or duration of the bouts, or both,

TABLE 4-5.
Activity programs, in ascending order of intensity, working from lowest to optimal level of fitness.

ACTIVITY	LEVEL[b]	DISTANCE	RATE	BOUTS PER DAY	TIME PER DAY	TIMES PER WEEK	COMMENTS
Walking	(LL):	1 mi.	1 mi:15 min.	1	15-17 min.	5	
	(OL):	3 mi.	1 mi:13 min.	1	38-43 min.	5	
		or					
		4 mi.	1 mi:13 min.	1	52-57 min.	4	
		or					
		5 mi.	1 mi:13 min.	1	62-67 min.	3	More detailed program, see Cooper, 1968.
Handball, Basketball, Tennis, Squash, or Badminton	(LL):		Continuous	1	10 min.	5[a]	Singles
	(OL):		Continuous	1	60 min.	3	Singles
			Continuous	1	45 min.	4	Singles
							More detailed program, see Cooper, 1968.
Combination Jogging & Walking	(LL):			1	30 min.	3	Walk, jog, walk, run, walk
	(OL):			1	30 min.	3	Walk, run, walk, sprint, walk
	alternate program:						
	(LL):	½ mi.	120 steps/min.	1		5	Walk
	(OL):	1 mi.		1		5	Jog and run alternately.
	or						
	(LL):	1 mi.	120 steps/min.	1		5	Walk
	(OL):	3 mi.		1		5	Jog and run alternately. More detailed programs, see *Adult Physical Fitness*, 1963; Bowerman & Harris, 1967; Cooper, 1968; The Healthy Life, 1966.
Cycling	(LL):	1 mi.	12 m.p.h.	1	5 min.	5	Stationary cycle equivalent
	(OL):	8 mi.	20 m.p.h.	1	25 min.	3-4	More detailed program, see Cooper, 1968.

Activity						Notes
Swimming	(LL):	25 yds,	25 yds.:35 sec.	4	2½ min. plus	5[a]	Rest between bouts variable.
		100 yds,	100 yds.:2½ min.	1	2½ min.	5	Continuous
			(progress in 100-yd. increments)				More detailed program, see *Adult Physical Fitness*, 1963; Cooper, 1968.
	(OL):	1000 yds.	100 yds.:2 min.	1	approx. 20 min.	3-4	Continuous
Running:							
Stationary:	(LL):		70-80 steps/min.	1	1 min.	5[a]	Continuous
	(OL):		80-90 steps/min.	1	20 min.	3-4	More detailed program, see *Adult Physical Fitness*, 1963; Cooper, 1968.
Forward:	(LL):	1 mi.		1	approx. 13 min.	5[a]	Walking
		1 mi.		1	approx. 11 min.	5	Alternate walk/run
		1 mi.		1	approx. 9½ min.	5	Run
	(OL):	2 mi.	1 mi:8½ min.	1	approx. 17 min.	3	More detailed programs, Cooper, 1968.
Bench-Stepping	(LL):	8" bench	120 counts/min. (30 steps/min.)	1	3 min.	5[a]	
	(OL):	15-18" bench	120 counts/min.	1	5 min.	3-4	More detailed program, Ricci, 1966.
Rope-Skipping (See Fig. 4-3)	(LL):			2	(½)(1)(½)(min.)	5[a]	Skip, rest, skip.
				3	(½)(1)(1)(½)(min.)	5	Skip, rest, skip, rest, skip.
			(gradual progression)				
	(OL):			2	(2)(½)(2)(min.)	5	Alternate skip, rest.
				3	(2)(½)(2)(2)(min.)	5	Alternate skip, rest.
				1	4-5 min.	3-4	Continuous
				1	6 min.	3-4	Continuous
							More detailed program see Baker, 1968; Jones et al, 1962; Ricci, 1966.
Combination	For variety, two or more activities can be alternated.						

[a] 3 times per week for these activities for first week or two.

[b] Progress from (LL): Lowest Fitness level, to (OL): Optimal or ideal fitness level

while decreasing the time interval for rest, so that eventually high intensity and duration can be accomplished with no actual rest periods.

The concept of interval training can very easily be applied to stationary bicycling, swimming, stationary and forward running, bench stepping, and rope skipping. Interval training has even been used successfully in rehabilitating cardiac patients. Interval training may be very simple, but can also become very complex when utilized for training purposes for track and swimming events. The program for rope skipping outlined in Table 4-5 is an example of a simplified type of interval training; two other examples of simple interval training methods are running and swimming.

For running you might initially select as your goal a six-minute mile. To interval train, you could run eight units of 220 yards, jogging so that you complete the 220 in 40 seconds with a three minute rest interval between each 220. You could gradually reduce the unit time to 30 seconds per 220 yard run, then gradually reduce the rest interval to one minute; then increase the unit to four-75 second 440 yard runs separated by three minutes rest; and so on until you have put together the six-minute mile.

After attaining the ability to swim at a moderate pace for 15 consecutive minutes, you could swim 25 yards at about 3/4 speed, get out of the water and walk back to the other side of the pool and repeat as many times as possible up to 20. Gradually increase speed, then gradually decrease rest interval if greater intensity and duration are desired.

The concept of interval training also has application to other kinds of conditioning, especially to muscular endurance improvement.

STRENGTH: ISOTONIC

Tests

Isotonic strength is tested by determining the greatest resistance (weight) a given muscle group can overcome by moving it through the full range of joint motion. Barbells are usually used and some rest between attempts, to reduce the effect of fatigue, is essential.

For example, to test the isotonic strength of the muscle groups involved in elbow flexion, you might use the arm curl test. Follow the procedures outlined in Table 4-6. You can safely start with a barbell that weighs from 1/4 to 1/3 of your own weight. For example, if you weigh 160 pounds, you would start with 50 pounds. If you are able to curl this weight easily using *only* the arms, immediately try 60 pounds. When a given weight becomes difficult,

TABLE 4-6. Exercises[a]

EXERCISE	GRIP	INITIAL POSITION	INTERMEDIATE POSITION	FINAL POSITION	PRINCIPLE MOVEMENT	BODY REGIONS DEVELOPED
1. Arm curl	Reverse	Thigh rest	—	Chest rest	Arm flexion	Front of upper arms Front of forearm
2. Clean	Regular	Crouch	Squat Rest Split Rest	Chest rest	Leg extension	Upper and lower legs Back of hips
3. Standing press	Regular	Chest rest	—	Standing press	Arm extension	Shoulders, back, upper chest, back of upper arms
4. Jerk	Regular	Chest rest	Split Press	Standing press	Leg extension	Backs and inner sides of lower legs, upper legs, back of hips
5. Snatch	Regular	Crouch	Squat Rest Split Rest	Standing press	Leg extension	Anterior shoulder, upper chest, arm, upper legs
6. Standing leg dead lift	Reverse	Dead lift	—	Thigh rest	Back extension	Lower back and back of thighs
7. Bent rowing	Regular	Dead lift	—	—	Elbow flexion	Back, back of shoulders, front of upper arms
8. Standing arm pull-over	Reverse	Pull-over	—	Standing press	Elbow extension	Front of chest, sides of chest, below arms, back of upper arms
9. Shoulder shrug	Regular	Thigh rest	—	—	Shoulders elevated	Upper shoulder, sides of neck
10. Squats or deep knee bends	Regular	Shoulder rest	—	Shoulder squat	Knee flexion	Legs

[a]Adapted from Massey, et al., 1959.

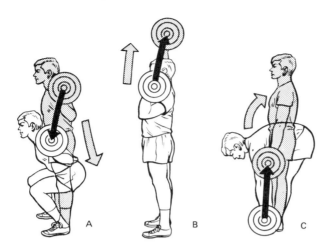

FIGURE 4-4. Examples of weight training exercises. (A) Squat; (B) standing press; (C) dead lift

then additional time is needed before the next lift. It may even be necessary to wait until another day and start fresh with the next weight. At the upper range it may be best to change to five pound increments. Average for the arm curl for college men is 75 pounds, for college women, 42 pounds. A better rule of thumb is that 80 pounds below your body weight is a little better than average for this test.

Another common isotonic strength test is the military or standing press. Following the procedures in Table 4-6, work through the same steps outlined for the arm curl to determine your maximum isotonic arm extension strength in this position. The ability to press a weight equal to one's own body weight is considered superior for men and one half the body weight is average.

General Principles of Improving Isotonic Strength

1. A demand must be placed on the specific muscles you wish to improve.

2. A smaller man will usually lift more, in proportion to his body size, than will a larger man.

3. The position for initiating the greatest force is one in which the muscle is slightly stretched.

4. Gains in strength and muscle size as a result of progressive loading will continue at a lower rate as training progresses.

5. The beginning weight trainer should begin with light weights to permit his body to adapt to the particular loaded movement.

6. Three sets (separated by adequate rest), progressing from three to nine repetitions per set, are the best for improving strength (Berger, 1962). After reaching nine repetitions, add weight so that fewer repetitions are possible and work up to nine again.

7. Each exercise should be carried through the full range of movement of the joint in order to keep the joint flexible.

8. Alternate work and rest days.

9. Strength is related to age and sex. Strength scores increase rapidly from twelve to nineteen years of age at a rate approximately proportional to body weight increase (Morehouse and Miller, 1963).

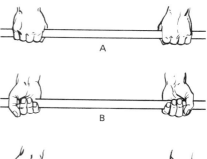

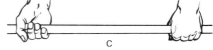

FIGURE 4-5. Grips used in weight training. (A) Regular or pronated; (B) reverse or supinated; (C) combination or alternate

Basic Approaches to Weight Training

Grips (see Fig. 4-5)

1. Regular or pronated (Fig. 4-5a)
2. Reverse or supinated (Fig. 4-5b)
3. Combination or alternate (Fig. 4-5c)

Body Positions

1. Crouch—bar on floor, knees fully flexed, regular grip
2. Deadlift—bar on floor, knees straight, regular grip or combination grip
3. Squat rest—bar at chest, knees fully flexed and parallel, regular grip

4. Split rest—bar at chest, legs split, regular grip

5. Shoulder squat—bar behind neck, knees flexed and parallel, regular grip

6. Thigh rest—bar on thighs, body erect, and regular or reverse grip

7. Chest rest—bar at chest, body erect, regular grip

8. Shoulder rest—bar behind neck, body erect, regular grip

9. Pull-over—bar on floor, body supine, regular grip

10. Squat press—bar overhead, body erect, regular grip

11. Split press—bar overhead, legs split, regular grip

12. Standing press—bar overhead, knees straight and parallel, regular grip

Movements (see Figure 4-10.)

1. Flexion (decreasing the angle of a joint, for example, bending elbow)

2. Extension (increasing the angle of a joint, for example, straightening elbow)

3. Rotation (for example, at shoulder; see Figure 4-10)

4. Abduction (movement away from body)

5. Adduction (movement toward body)

Basic Exercises (see Table 4-6 and Figure 4-4)

Standard Equipment
Barbell with sleeves or collars: 5-8' long; 1" in diameter; 25 pounds (5-foot bar with collars); 30 pounds (6-foot bar with collars). Assorted weighted plates or discs: 1¼, 2½, 5, 7½, 10, 15, 20, 25, 35, 45, 75, and 100 pounds.
Bench: 10" wide; 18" high; minimum 3' in length.

Programs

(If you desire more specific directions, see Massey et al., 1959; Murray & Karpovich, 1957; O'Shea, 1969; Rasch, 1966.)
The fraction beside each exercise indicates the ratio of the weight of the barbell to body weight recommended for the first workout.

Arm curl (1/4)
Military or standing press (1/3)
Pull-over on bench (1/10)
Bent over rowing (1/2)
Straight leg dead left (1/2)
Supine press on bench (1/2)
Squats or deep knee bends (1/2)

Minimum recommended repetitions is 3 each for 3 sets. When 9 to 12 repetitions are achieved, increase the barbell weight by 5 pounds (lower body) or 2½ pounds (upper body) for that exercise in the next training period. Progress to 9 or 12 again, then add weight again. Record daily repetitions and weight adjustments carefully.

ISOMETRIC STRENGTH

Tests

In order to test isometric strength, some type of gauge is needed to measure force exerted. Strain gauges for cables and dynamometers are commonly used. (For detailed tests of many muscle groups, see Clarke, Bailey, and Shea, 1952; Clark, 1957.)

Grip strength. (Equipment: spring type grip dynamometer.) Squeeze the dynamometer with maximal effort, with the arm and hand away from the body. This test may provide some indication of the total body strength. Norms for men: superior, 170—145 pounds; average, 135—100; deficient, 90—75 pounds (Murray and Karpovich, 1957). Average for college women, 65 pounds.

Back extension strength. (Equipment: (1) cable tensiometer, an instrument designed to measure the tension of aircraft control cable. Cable tension is determined from the force needed to create offset on a riser in a cable stretched between two set points. This tension is converted into pounds on a calibration chart. (2) Standard back and leg spring dynamometer.) Alternate bar grip (see Fig. 4-5), knees locked, then lean and pull backward. Norms for men: superior, 520—460 pounds; average, 400—280 pounds; deficient, 220—160 pounds (Massey et al., 1959).

Leg extension strength. (Equipment: cable tensiometer or back and leg dynamometer.) The bar rests on the upper legs; using regular grip (see Fig. 4-5), extend legs against resistance. Norms for men: superior, 875—750 pounds; average, 625—375 pounds; deficient, 250—125 pounds (Massey et al., 1959).

General Principles

1. Holding the isometric contraction for longer than 6 seconds results in greater strength gains; 10—12 seconds is recommended.

2. Repetitive isometric exercises produce an increase in isometric strength

significantly higher than that from the single isometric exercise routine (Meyers, 1967).

3. The intensity of single contractions seems to be of greater importance than the frequency with which these single contractions are performed (Morehouse, 1967).

4. Repeating a short maximal contraction several times a day does not increase the training effect (Royce, 1964).

5. Differences in individual responses indicate that not all individuals possess the same physiological capacity to benefit from isometric training (Jones, 1968).

6. Improperly conducted isometric programs can result in limitations of range of motion and reduced joint flexibility.

7. The greatest value of isometric training is the development of strength at a specific point (or points, if more than one is utilized in training). It may also be useful for increasing strength so that muscular endurance exercises can be undertaken.

Methods

1. Make sure that muscle action is vigorous and near maximum level.

2. Hold the contraction for 10 seconds, using two sets daily.

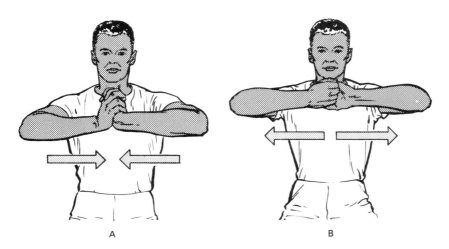

A   B

FIGURE 4-6. Examples of isometric exercises without equipment

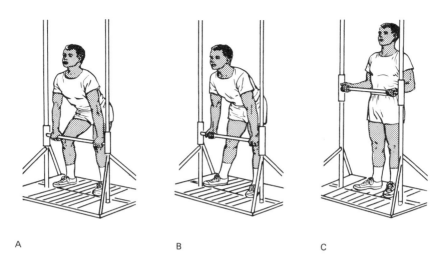

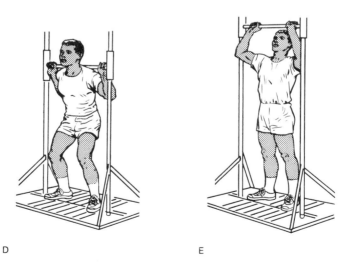

FIGURE 4-7. Weight training exercises used as isometric exercises. (A) Bent knee middle pull; (B) straight leg middle pull; (C) curl; (D) high squat; (E) middle press

3. Perform five days per week.

4. Include a variety of isometric exercises to insure development of strength in all the major parts of the body.

5. Use more than one point in the full range of motion of a joint. (See principles 6 and 7, page 42.)

Programs

Using a towel, rope, or fixed bar, or even with no equipment, you can perform the following types of isometric actions (see Fig. 4-6):
a. Push in with hands together.
b. Pull up on fixed object.
c. Press out to side against wall.
d. Pull head back against hands.
e. Press up on immovable object.
f. Press down on fixed object.

Most weight training exercises can also be done as isometric exercises (see Fig. 4-7); for example:
a. High press
b. Upright row
c. Two-hand curl
d. Low squat
e. Low pull

(For more specific directions, see *Adult Physical Fitness*, 1963; O'Shea, 1969; Steinhaus, 1957.)

MUSCULAR ENDURANCE

Tests

Muscular endurance is assessed by working against a resistance representing less than one's maximal strength. *Isometric* endurance involves holding a contraction against a fixed resistance or in a fixed position for as long as possible (example: holding books out to the side at arm's length). *Isotonic* endurance is tested with weights (a specific weight or a specific percentage of the individual's maximum) or by using the person's own body weight as the resistance (pull-ups, push-ups, sit-ups, and so on). Two factors greatly affect test results: (1) percentage of maximum force being used, and (2) rate of repetitions (slower rate=greater endurance in some tests). In all isotonic tests, a standardized rate is essential for comparative purposes.

Pull-up test for men. Using a horizontal bar, hang from the bar with forward or reverse grip (palms facing away from or toward you), hands at shoulder width. Pull up with arms, without swinging body, until chin is above the level of the bar; lower body until arms are fully extended; repeat as many times as possible. Average for college-age men: 8.

Push-up test for men. Assume a prone position, keeping the back straight, arms bent so that the hands are placed on the floor just under the shoulders; push up from the floor to the front leaning rest position, return to the prone position, touching only the chest each time. Repeat as many times as possible. Average for college-age men: 25.

Sit-up test. Assume a supine position, knees bent so that heels are 8-10" from buttocks, hands locked behind the neck or head. Partner holds feet. Curl the trunk, with lower back flat, to flexed position, touch chest to upper legs, return to supine position, and repeat as often as possible. May be done with time limit or at a given rate. Averages: college-age men, 40; college-age women, 20.

Bar dips test for men (Fig. 4-8). (Equipment: dipping bars or parallel bars.) Jump to bars in front support position; lower body until the angle of the upper arm and forearm is slightly less than a right angle; push up to the straight arm position and repeat as often as possible. Average for college-age males: 9.

Modified push-up test for women (Clarke, 1957). (Equipment: stall bar

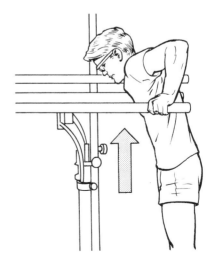

FIGURE 4-8. Bar dip test of muscular endurance (for men)

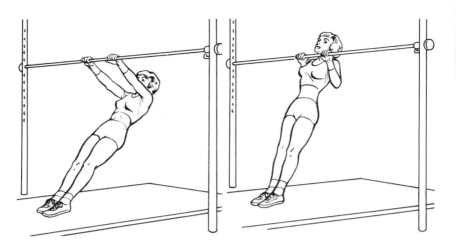

FIGURE 4-9. Modified pull-up test (for women)

bench or a stool 13" high.) Grasp the outer edges of the bench, assuming a front-leaning rest position; lower the body so that the upper chest touches the near edge of the bench, and return to the starting position, repeating as many times as possible. Average for college-age women: 18.

Modified pull-up test for women (Clarke, 1957). (Equipment: adjustable horizontal bar, adjusted to chest height.) Grasp the bar with regular (forward) grip (Fig. 4-9); slide feet under the bar until the body and arms form approximately a right angle and the weight is supported by the heels; pull up chest to the bar and return to starting position; repeat as many times as possible. Average for college-age women: 25.

General Principles

1. A demand to persist and repeat must be placed on the specific muscles you wish to improve.

2. Isotonic endurance involves repetition of the same isotonic movement with some manipulation of load (at less than maximum) or rate of execution.

3. Isometric endurance involves varying the force of muscular contraction from maximum to a percentage of maximum in a continual holding of an isometric contraction (Kroll, 1966).

4. Strong muscles fatigue more rapidly than weak muscles but maintain a higher level of absolute strength throughout the fatigue process.

5. Higher levels of strength generally provide for the capacity to maintain greater isometric force with slower onset of fatigue and also provide for greater isotonic endurance at a given load.

6. Isotonic endurance or isometric endurance at a specific percentage of the individual's maximum force is generally related not to the individual's strength, but to the specific percentage of maximum.

7. Soreness will result initially (about 24 hours after first exercise), but you may minimize it by starting at an easy load with low repetitions and working up gradually.

Methods

1. For general improvement, work on all major body areas.
   a. Arms and shoulders
   b. Abdominals and back
   c. Legs
2. Extend repetitions with each session.
3. It is possible to use weights to overload a movement as well as the resistance of your own body weight. When using weights, adjust the load so that the number of repetitions will be no less than 15.
4. Rotate exercises so as not to overextend a particular muscle group all at once.
5. A small sand bag or a weight without the bar may be used to increase the load for sit-ups. Small amounts of weight can also be added by various means to add to the load in pull-ups and push-ups.
6. When one repetition of a given exercise (for example, pull-ups) cannot be accomplished, the strength of that muscle group is probably less than the resistance furnished by the body. The strength must be increased first, preferably by isotonic strength training or, if strength level is close to that required, eccentric or isometric exercise may help. (For example, use any method of getting to the "up" position on the chinning bar and either hold yourself up (isometric contraction) or gradually lower yourself (eccentric contraction.)

Programs

Examples of calisthenic-type activities (Casady, 1965).
Abdominal curl: assume supine position on the floor; curl upper trunk and head upward and forward while keeping lower back in contact with the floor, slowly lower upper trunk to floor.

Sit-ups with bent legs.

Sit-up and leg raise: assume supine position on the floor with hands by sides and legs extended; sit up and raise legs at the same time and touch feet with hands while balancing on buttocks; return to starting position.

Push-ups.

Modified push-ups.

Squat thrust with push-up: assume standing position; squat; place hands on the floor outside feet, with support on extended arms; thrust feet backward, taking front leaning rest position; perform a push-up; return to squat position; return to standing position and repeat.

(Specific muscular endurance programs may be found in Massey et al., 1959; O'Shea, 1969; Rasch, 1966.)

Activities using equipment.

Hanging-type activities

1. Rope climbing
2. Pegboard climbing. Holes are spaced 6–15" apart, 1–1½" in diameter. Pegs are 12" long and are inserted in the holes at a slight downward angle as individual uses peg placement to climb upward.
3. Overhead ladder
   a. Travel on one rail.
   b. Travel on both rails.
   c. Travel on rungs of ladder.
4. Parallel bar
   a. Perform dips (Fig. 4-8).
   b. Travel length of bars, using short alternate arm movements.
   c. "Hop" length of bars, using arms.
5. Horizontal Bar
   a. Do pull-ups.
   b. Do modified pull-ups (low bar).
   c. Perform double leg raise, knees bent or knees straight.
      1) To horizontal position with legs
      2) Toes to bar

Weight Lifting

Perform the exercises listed in the isotonic strength section using a base of 15 or more repetitions. Most muscle groups can be extra-loaded with weights.

FLEXIBILITY

Tests

There is no single test that provides adequate information about the flexibility of all the major joints of the body. One may have excellent trunk flexibility, for example, but very poor hip and trunk extensibility. The two most common tests of flexibility and normal ranges of motion for the major joints of the body are illustrated in Fig. 4-10.

General Priniciples

1. Demand for full extension, flexion, or both must be placed on the joint. This means that muscles and tendons must be gradually accustomed to additional stretch.

2. Stretch gently. In forcing extension or flexion of a joint, do so very gently and gradually. This will help prevent excess stretch and possible tissue damage.

3. Practice regularly. Only faithful adherence to a regular schedule will provide any significant improvement in flexibility.

Methods and Programs

Little is known about the minimum requirement for producing gains in flexibility, but practical experience has shown that flexibility improvement is most likely to result from distributed rather than massed efforts. That is, it is apparently better to do three sets of 10 stretches morning, noon, and evening, than to do 30 all at once. We recommend a minimum of ten "stretch demands" per day for each specific flexibility you wish to improve, at least five days per week, until the range of motion you desire has been attained. Then 10 per day for each specific flexibility, three days per week, is probably adequate.

The most important specific flexibilities probably are neck and shoulder flexibility, back extension, and hip flexion (with knees straight to stretch the hamstrings). Individuals participating in vigorous sports activity may also find it advantageous to improve especially the extensibility of the elbow, wrist, knee, and ankle joints.

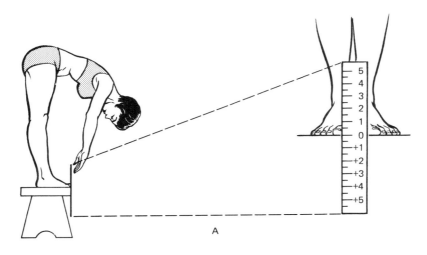

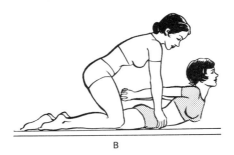

FIGURE 4-10. Flexibility tests. (A) Trunk flexion; score in inches, plus below line, minus above line; average for college men +1", for college women + 3.5". (B) Trunk extension; score in inches; average for college men 12", for college women 18". (C) Normal range of motion in selected joints.

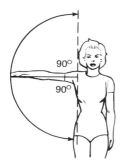
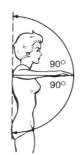
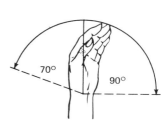

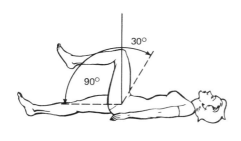
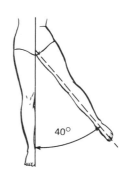

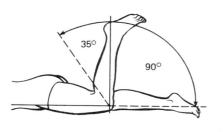
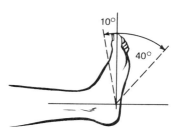

C

BODY COMPOSITION

Tests

Two reasonably accurate laboratory methods are commonly used today for estimating body fat (that is, the percentage of the total body composition that is fat tissue.) Both of these require some instruments. One is a skin-fold thickness method for estimating percent of body fat and the second is a body density or underwater weighing method. The former involves the use of a skinfold caliper, which is designed to eliminate as much as possible any variability introduced by the examiner. The body density method involves a water tank, suspensory equipment for lowering the individual into the water, a reasonably sensitive scale, and a means for determining the residual lung volume (the amount of air trapped in the lungs, which cannot be exhaled even with a forceful expiration). Norm: anything above 14 percent for men or 20 percent for women should be considered excess fat (Johnson, 1966). Many college departments of physical education, health education, or nutrition have available one or both of these types of equipment. You can also purchase an excellent and reliable skinfold caliper for approximately $70.[1] Over the years, this may be a wise investment.

The second-best approach to determining ideal body weight and excess body fat is the use of the Willoughby method (McGavack, 1965; Willoughby, 1932) for determining optimal body weight. A good tape measure, a good sliding wooden caliper, and the formula and its accompanying table are the essential tools. Since the sliding wooden caliper is a rather specialized piece of equipment, though inexpensive, this method has not been reproduced here. If you are interested in using this method, see Johnson et al., (1966).

If none of the foregoing methods is practical for you, we suggest that you use two simpler methods in combination. The standard height-weight table (Appendix B) may be used along with the Overweight Index. (Fabry et al., 1964; Johnson et al. 1966):

OW Index = 100 X body weight (kilograms) ÷ height (centimeters) − 100

With the OW Index, anything in excess of 110 percent represents obesity. Agreement between the standard height-weight table and the Overweight Index provides some evidence concerning normal or excess body fat.

[1]Write to J. A. Preston Corp., 71 Fifth Avenue, New York, N.Y. 10003 for information.

General Principles

To control or reduce the amount of fat stored in the body, you should find the following scientific principles helpful.

The diet should be composed of the proper food in the proper proportions (see Chapter 11). Excess fat intake (especially of *saturated fat*) and excessive simple sugar intake should be especially avoided ("Present Knowledge of Carbohydrates," 1966; "Present Knowledge of Fat," 1966). If a complete nutrient analysis is not practical, you can cut out or cut down on the following foods: dairy and meat fats (drink skim milk; eliminate pork, bacon, and sausage; trim the fat from meats that you do eat), cakes and pies, and ice cream. Use only vegetable oils in cooking and eliminate as much as possible commercially prepared products that do not use vegetable shortening.

Eat the proper amount of food. You will gain weight, usually in the form of excess body fat, if you consume more calories than you expend per day. Conversely, excess body fat cannot be eliminated unless fewer calories are consumed than are expended. In gaining or losing weight, about 3500 calories equal one pound (Wishnofsky, 1958).

Spread the caloric intake evenly over at least three meals per day. There is some evidence that "gorging," that is, taking in all calories at one or two sittings per day, has a tendency to promote obesity and raise blood cholesterol levels (Fabry et al., 1964; Johnson and Cooper, 1967).

Make sure that you engage in adequate amounts of daily physical activity, whether as part of your occupation or through purposeful and regularly scheduled exercise. Adequate amounts of daily physical activity have been demonstrated to contribute to weight maintenance or reduction in at least three ways: (1) The increase in caloric expenditure, though not dramatic in moderate and less strenuous activities (Fig. 4-11), nevertheless contributes to a favorable balance between caloric intake and caloric expenditure; (2) regular physical activity apparently assists the appestat, located in the hypothalamus, to keep appetite in line with actual body needs, thus contributing to a more favorable caloric balance (Mayer, 1960); (3) regular and reasonably vigorous physical activity contributes to a more favorable body composition, that is, a lower percentage of body fat, even for a given body weight (Jones et al., 1964; Parizkova and Stankova, 1964; Wikander and Johnson, n.d.). (Fig. 4-12). Most of the evidence indicates that spot reducing, that is, exercising a particular area of the body to cause removal of fat deposits from that area, is no more effective than more generalized exercise (Johnson et al., 1966).

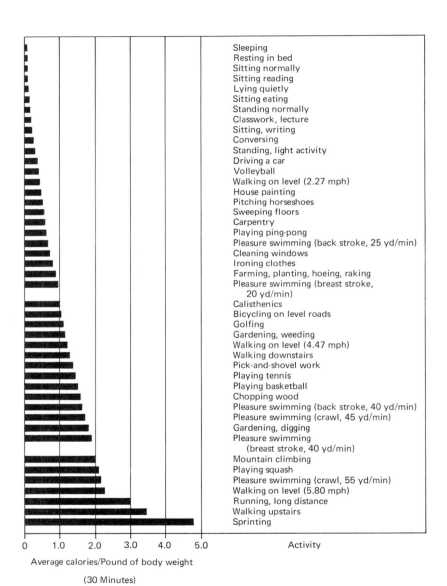

FIGURE 4-11. Calorie expenditure in various daily activities

do a complete knee bend and then return to the standing position; with only one foot on the beam do a complete squat and return to the standing position (do not try this with a weak or damaged knee). Most college-age men and women can score at least 8 points on this test.

6. With your finger touching a specific point on the floor, walk around it in a circle 10 times in 30 seconds. Then attempt to walk a straight line for 10' within a 5-second period (*The Healthy Life*, 1966).

General Principles

The following general principles apply to balance improvement.

1. Demand must be placed upon the systems involved (primarily sensory, perceptual, and neuromuscular).

2. Repetition is necessary; the whole method is probably best; distributed practice is best; mental practice may help; speed should be sacrificed for accuracy when necessary.

3. It may be helpful to overload the senses for balance improvement, for example, by closing the eyes or adding weights in a particular way to throw the body off balance.

4. Attempt to improve balance in as many different positions and in as many different kinds of movement as possible.

Methods and Programs

There are no specific programs for improving general balance. As mentioned above, each kind of balance apparently is independent of the other. We recommend that any person interested in improving general balance should undertake a program of some regularity in which he simply works at improving his performance on the tests described above, in addition to as many other positions and activities as he can invent.

AGILITY

Tests

Two tests of agility are illustrated in Fig. 5-1. Another simple test, the sidestepping test, is scored by determining the number of complete trips made by shuffling sideways as quickly as possible between two lines placed 8' apart on the floor during a 10 second period. Average score is 6.

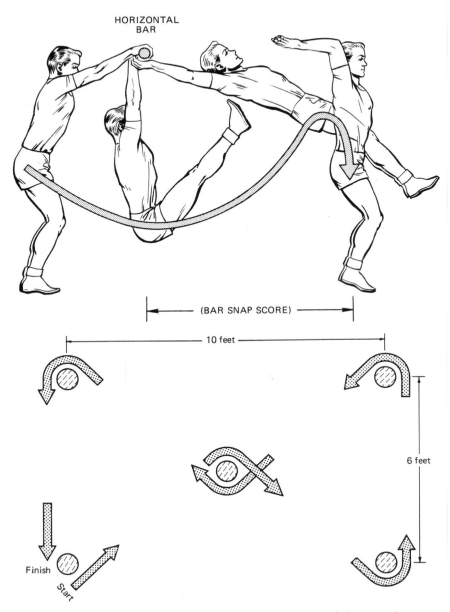

FIGURE 5-1. Agility tests. (A) Average for college men 5'0"; (B) average for college men, 8.0 seconds, for college women 12.0 seconds

General Principles

The following principles are important for improvement in agility.

1. Demand must be placed upon the systems involved.

2. Repetition is essential; the whole method will most often be the best method. Distributed practice is best; pushing too far beyond the point of fatigue may be detrimental to learning; accuracy and speed must be combined in equal amounts unless it is absolutely impossible to move accurately at higher speeds.

3. It is unlikely that agility of one kind concomitantly improves every kind of agility. Therefore, if you want to develop a specific kind of agility, practice that one.

Methods and Programs

The only way to improve a specific kind of agility is to practice it, whether it is one of the tests illustrated in Fig. 5-1 or one of the much more specific kinds of movements in sports.

POWER

Testing

In general, power can be tested by measuring performance of explosive movement.

Leg power.
Vertical jump (see Fig. 5-2).
The standing broad jump may also be used. Average for college-age men is 7'3", for college-age women, 5'0".

Arm and shoulder power.
Softball distance throw. Throw for distance, standardizing the approach to the restraining line. Average for 12" ball: for men, 165'; for women, 85'.
Medicine ball put. (Equipment: 12 pound medicine ball) "Put," do not "throw" the ball (shove the ball forward and upward at about a 45° angle from the shoulder), standardizing preliminary approaching movement. Average for college-age men: 35'.

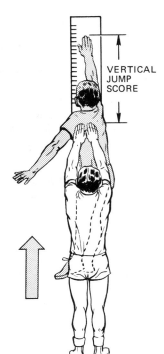

FIGURE 5-2. Vertical jump; average for college men 20″, for college women 13″

General Principles

1. Basically, the rate of working must be increased, the force of application increased, or both.

2. Power depends a great deal upon neuromuscular coordination.

3. Mechanical efficiency is a prime factor.

4. Motivation and previous experience can modify central nervous system inhibition, which influences power development.

5. Improvement in isotonic strength is more highly related to power improvement than is isometric strength improvement (Berger and Bluschke, 1967).

Methods

1. Practice specific movement at normal speed and use weights for overload when overload is feasible. Thus the power movement, not strength alone, is emphasized in training.

2. Improve your technique to minimize unnecessary and unrelated movement.

3. Understand and use the mechanical principles related to the movement.

SPEED AND MOVEMENT TIME

Tests

Tests for speed (total time lapse for movement of the body from one point to another) generally take the form of a "dash" of some 50 to 220 yards. Average for college-age men (50 yards) is 6.8 seconds; for college women, 8.2 seconds. Unfortunately, reaction time in starting considerably affects time in the shorter dashes, and unfit persons cannot maintain all-out effort in the longer dashes where reaction time is not quite so critical. One solution is to time the person at his maximum speed from the 20-yard mark to the 60-yard mark in a 60-yard dash, thus measuring true maximal running speed without the effect of the starting reaction time and the effects of the mechanics of the start.

Movement time (movement of isolated body parts) can only be measured with a sensitive timing device (as with reaction time).

General Principles

1. A demand must be made on the specific movement(s).

2. Weight training does not necessarily result in muscular tightness and in a decrease of muscular contraction speed (Capen, 1950; Wilkins, 1952).

3. Urging a person to move more rapidly will increase his speed of movement, but may well decrease accuracy (Morehouse and Miller, 1963).

4. Total body running speed and reaction time are independent of each other, as are reaction time and movement time.

5. In skills in which speed is the predominant factor for successful performance, the most efficient results are attained by early emphasis on speed (Solley, 1952).

6. Overloading the movements may cause a feeling of increased speed after the load is removed, but does not necessarily cause an actual increase in speed of movement. However such training may shorten movement time.

Methods and Programs

The only way to increase running speed or speed of movement is to work at the movement or at the running. Remember that dash time reflects some endurance, in that you must repeat the driving movements until past the finish line, so that to some extent improving "power endurance" may help improve absolute speed. Reaction time and skill in starting are also very critical factors.

Strength increase may aid speed somewhat, but the use of "spats" (weighted anklets) and weighted vests to improve running speed is of dubious value (Anderson, 1961).

Overloading a body part's movement in regular training may bring about quicker movement time.

REACTION TIME

Testing

Reaction time is best evaluated by means of some device in which a signal initiates an electric timer (graduated in divisions of 1/100 or 1/1000 of a second) and the beginning of the person's response stops the timer. Mechanical devices, which take advantage of the known rate of an object's fall due to gravity, have also been devised for testing reaction time. Reaction time is generally quickest when it involves smaller, finer muscles (such as those used for pushing a button with the thumb, as contrasted with initiating a jump from a mat), and is quicker in response to tactile or sound stimuli than to visual stimuli (Singer, 1968). Reaction time tends to be slower in the aged and is often affected adversely by fatigue of the muscles involved (Singer, 1968). Athletes or people who are required to act quickly usually have quicker reaction times than others do (Singer, 1968).

Men react faster than women, and both sexes react most quickly between the ages of 21 and 30 (Morehouse and Miller, 1963). There are great individual differences among persons, and the reaction time to all kinds of stimuli will be lengthened if the stimuli are complicated (Morehouse and Miller, 1963). Small-muscle reaction time, as measured by pressing a button with the thumb, averages .16 second in college men and .17 second in college women.

GENERAL PRINCIPLES

1. "Demand" is essential.

2. Regularity of practice is essential.

3. Certain persons will probably never be able to become extremely quick in reaction; other persons, who never practice a given response, may always be quicker.

Methods and Programs

1. Practice often and in a variety of ways if you wish to improve general reaction time.

2. Overload by complicating stimuli, making the response more complex (for example, choice reaction time such as involved in sorting playing cards by suit; responding to a red light with one hand, a white light with the other, and so on.).

3. Many enjoyable and interesting little games and contests can be invented as aids to improving reaction time. Many will also involve total response time, but still include reaction time. (Examples: hand-slapping, in which an opponent places hands palms up several inches apart, and you place palms down on his palms; when he moves to rotate hands and tries to slap your hands on top, you react by moving your hands away. Another game is catching a ruler between your thumb and forefinger when released by another person so that it is even with your finger and thumb at release. Try removing the hand from a surface when a marble or coin is dropped from above, gradually reducing distance of marble above hand; and so on).

YOU SHOULD NOW UNDERSTAND:

That specific kinds of motor ability may be difficult to improve.

That one kind of motor performance does not necessarily carry over to other kinds (for example, speed to agility).

That even within one kind of motor performance, transfer is not automatic (for example, two kinds of agility tests).

That many of the principles for improving the various kinds of motor ability are empirically or logically derived and may or may not lead to significent improvement.

How to test for specific kinds of motor abilities.

6

THE IDEAL CHALLENGE
a personalized
general fitness approach

The purpose of this chapter is to help you:
1. Understand the principles of general physical fitness
   attainment, especially via circuit training
2. Know how to set up and participate
   in a circuit-training program

THE PHYSICAL FITNESS PROGRAM

We have described physical fitness and motor ability tests with which you can evaluate your status, general principles for improvement, and examples of activities and programs that may bring about improvement. We want to emphasize at this point that the ideal program for those not interested in achieving specific competitive sports goals is a *general physical fitness program*, emphasizing cardiovascular health and aimed at improving the other fitness and motor ability qualities, based on the individual's needs. The basic format of such a program is suggested in Chapters 4 and 5.

Calisthenic and rhythmic exercise programs are certainly of some value, but do not usually produce significant improvement in general fitness qualities because, in general, demand is not sufficient.

Weight lifting and body building programs can improve strength and muscular endurance, but they are all too often undertaken with indifference toward health goals and with the immature belief that strength and physique are important for social acceptance. The fact that one can be assured of an improved physique often leads the individual away from the important health goals, especially the very important cardiovascular fitness. It is our firm belief that the ideal general physical fitness program is one that focuses upon circulo-respiratory fitness, but does take into account the need for improving or maintaining minimal levels of strength, muscular endurance, flexibility, and optimal body composition. These latter aspects of physical fitness, as well as improvement of motor ability, may be handled according to your interests and experience, the available facilities and equipment, and most important, your deficiencies. Such a balanced general physical fitness program can be achieved in many ways. You can simply work on each individual fitness quality in any scientifically sound manner. We suggest that you consider the concept of circuit training, which combines all fitness elements in a systematic way, if you wish to adopt a general physical fitness program that is well balanced and yet provides some escape from boredom. A chief advantage of circuit training is regular and ongoing evaluation, which is built into the program.

Circuit training can provide vigorous activity in a number of selected fitness and motor ability activities and is aimed at developing all the basic physical fitness components, performed in an interesting and imaginative fashion. The individual works on each activity within the circuit, and within his individual capacity attempts to complete the prescribed circuit within a specified time limit. He records his own results and progress. Progress is achieved by reduction in time, by an increase in the number of repetitions of each individual exercise, and by increasing the demand or load at each station within the circuit. Some advantages of circuit training are: (1) A large number of persons can be accommodated at the same time, (2) the individual works at his own rate within his own capacity, (3) the goals are both immediately obtainable and easily evaluated, and (4) "target time," the attempt to complete the circuit in a certain maximum time, provides a strong motivational factor.

We have found it best to begin with a standard circuit, to progress to the second or third level, and then to individualize your circuit based on your particular interests and needs, always keeping in mind the importance of the circulo-respiratory fitness level. We offer two standard circuits, each with two levels of progression, one for men and one for women.

CIRCUIT TRAINING PROGRAM

The circuit we describe is designed to meet the conditioning needs of a heterogeneous group of students. It is adaptable to various facilities, using available equipment or no equipment, if time must be limited. Though the circuit is designed for use by larger groups, you can readily adapt it to your individual needs. The recommended circuit is based on these principles:

1. CR capacity determines the classification into one of four groups.

2. The lower the CR capacity, the higher the percentage of time assigned to the CR component and the warm-up component.

3. The time remaining is split between warm-up, flexibility, strength, and muscular endurance activities.

4. Repetitions are based on either an evaluation of the individual's maximum capacity or individual motivation.

5. Advancement to a new classification is based on a retest of CR capacity, using the basic CR test.

6. The group 4 classification provides individuality and is designed for the highly fit, those who need remedial work, and the handicapped, all of whom need a personalized circuit.

7. All participants will finish the circuit at the same time.

Test for CR Capacity

The 12-minute test (Cooper, 1968), as described on page 31, may be used for the initial classification and reclassification.

IF YOU COVER	YOU ARE IN GROUP
less than 1.24 miles	1
1.25 to 1.49 miles	2
1.50 to 1.74 miles	3
1.75 miles or more	4

If you do not know your 12-minute field test score and do not wish to take the test, assume classification 1.

CR Component for Men and Women

ACTIVITY	EQUIPMENT	REPS.
Jogging (and interspersed walking if necessary)	None	Number of laps (including parts of laps) or distance run in the allotted time.

Other components for men.

FLEXIBILITY AND MUSCULAR STRENGTH ACTIVITIES

ACTIVITY	EQUIPMENT	A REPS.	B REPS.
Toe Touch	None	10	20
Body Bender	None	10	15
Prone Arch	None	10	20
Sitting Stretch	None	10	15
Leg Raiser	None	5	10
Leg Raiser (on extended arm)	None	10	15
Flutter Kick	None	20	40

WARM-UP ACTIVITIES

ACTIVITY	EQUIPMENT	LEVEL A REPS.	LEVEL B REPS.
Side Straddle Hop	None	20	50
Squat Thrust	None	10	25
Squat Jump	None	20	50
Sit-up (arms extended, knees up)	None	15	30
Sprinter	None	20	50
Bench Step	Bench	10	25
Rope Jump	Rope	50	100

NECK, ARMS AND SHOULDERS: MUSCULAR STRENGTH AND ENDURANCE ACTIVITIES

ACTIVITY	EQUIPMENT	A REPS.	WEIGHT	B REPS.	WEIGHT
Push-up	None	50% max.		75% max.	
Pull-up	Horizontal bar	50% max.		75% max.	
Dip	Parallel bars	50% max.		75% max.	
Bench Press	Barbell	3-10	60#	3-15	80#
Two-arm Curl	Barbell	3-10	40#	3-15	50#
Two-arm Press	Barbell	3-10	50#	3-15	60#
Bent-over Rowing	Barbell	3-8	65#	3-10	85#
Wrist Roll	18" Handle, 24" Cord	1-5	15#	5-10	15#

TRUNK MUSCULAR STRENGTH AND ENDURANCE ACTIVITIES

ACTIVITY	EQUIPMENT	A REPS.	WEIGHT	B REPS.	WEIGHT
Bent Knee Sit-up	None	50% (1 min. max.)		75% (1 min. max.)	
Stiff Leg Dead Lift	Barbell	3-8	65#	3-10	85#
Side Bender	Barbell	3-8	50#	3-10	60#

LEG MUSCULAR STRENGTH-ENDURANCE ACTIVITIES

ACTIVITY	EQUIPMENT	A REPS.	WEIGHT	B REPS.	WEIGHT
Straddle Bench Jump	Bench (12") Dumbbells	3-10	25#	10-25	20#
3/4 Squat	Barbell	3-10	75#	3-15	95#

Other components for women. Warm-up activities same as listing for men. Flexibility-muscular strength activities same as listing for men.

NECK, ARMS AND SHOULDERS:
MUSCULAR STRENGTH AND ENDURANCE ACTIVITIES

ACTIVITY	EQUIPMENT	A REPS.	WEIGHT	B REPS.	WEIGHT
Modified Push-up	None	50% max.		75% max.	
Modified Pull-up	Parallel Bars	50% max.		75% max.	
Two-arm Curl	Dumbbells	3-10	30#	3-15	20#
Two-arm Press	Dumbbells	3-10	40#	3-15	30#
Wrist Roll	18" Handle, 24" Cord	1-5	5#	5-10	5#

TRUNK MUSCULAR STRENGTH AND ENDURANCE ACTIVITIES

ACTIVITY	EQUIPMENT	A REPS.	WEIGHT	B REPS.	WEIGHT
Bent Knee Sit-up	None	50% (1 min. max.)		75% (1 min. max.)	
Stiff Leg Dead Lift	Barbell	3-8	40#	3-10	50#

LEG MUSCULAR STRENGTH-ENDURANCE ACTIVITIES

ACTIVITY	EQUIPMENT	A REPS.	B REPS.
Straddle Bench Jump	Bench 8''-10''	3-10	10-25

COMPONENT TIME ASSIGNMENTS

LENGTH OF CIRCUIT (MINUTES)	CLASSI-FICATION	LENGTH OF CARDIO-VASCULAR COMPONENT (CV) (MINUTES)	LENGTH OF WARM-UP AND FLEXIBILITY (WF) COMPONENTS (MINUTES)	LENGTH OF STRENGTH COMPONENTS (SC)(MINUTES)
	1	5	5	0
	2	4	3	3
10	3	3	2	5
	4	3-7	1-2	2-7
	1	7	5	3
	2	6	4	5
15	3	5	3	7
	4	5-9	2-3	4-7
	1	9	5	6
	2	8	5	7
20	3	7	4	9
	4	7-10	2-4	6-11
	1	11	5	9
	2	10	5	10
25	3	9	5	11
	4	9-15	2-5	8-14
	1	13	5	12
	2	12	5	13
30	3	11	5	14
	4	11-18	2-5	10-17

STATION	COMPONENT
1	Warm-up, flexibility—muscular endurance
2	Warm-up, flexibility—muscular endurance
3	Warm-up, flexibility—muscular endurance
4	Muscular strength—endurance
5	Muscular strength—endurance
6	Muscular strength—endurance
7	Cardiovascular endurance

CLASSI- FICATION	CARDIO- VASCULAR	TIME WARM-UP AND FLEXIBILITY	STRENGTH COMPONENTS	STATION ROTATION
1	5	5	0	1-2-3-7
2	4	3	3	2-3-4-5-7
3	3	2	5	3-4-5-6-1-7
4	3-7	1-2	2-7	Arranged

The instructor or organizer assigns the activities for each station and encourages any personal selection within the station that seems reasonable. At the 5-minute circuit mark the classification 1 students immediately terminate the activity they are working on and begin jogging. Group 2 begins jogging at the 6-minute mark and group 3 begins jogging at the 7-minute mark. Each member of group 4, the individualized group, observes his own time.

Sample Individualized Record Sheet

Name_____John Doe_____.

Date	9/12						
CR Test Score (miles)	1.60						
Classification	3						

Date	9/10	9/10	9/10	9/10	9/10	
Time Tests	Push- up	Dip	Press	Sit-up	Straddle Jump	
Weight (pounds)			50		20	
Maximum Repetitions	12	8	6	50	15	

Circuit

Classification___3__

TIME	COMPONENT	NO.	ACTIVITY	REPETITIONS	WEIGHT
3	CV		Jogging		
2	WF	1	Squat thrust	20	
		2	Sprinter	20	
		3			
		4			
		5			
		6			
5	SE	1	Push-up	6	
		2	Dip	4	
		3	Two-arm Press	3-10	50
		4	Sit-up	25	
		5	Straddle Jump	10-25	20
		6			
		7			
		8			
		9			
		10			

Sample Daily Record Sheet

			ACTIVITY S AND E									
		CR	1	2	3	4	5	6	7	8	9	10
DATE	TIME (MINUTES)	DISTANCE (LAPS)	REPETITIONS (X—INDICATES NO CHANGE)									
9/17	3	12	x	x	4	x	15					
9/19	3	10½	x	x	x	x	x					
9/24	3	13	x	5	5	x	20					
9/26	3	12½	8	x	6	30	x					

Participants can record their own data by marking file cards or large wall charts. It is recommended that participants graph their progress periodically as an added incentive to improve. Other circuits may be developed and others may be found in Hakes and Rosemeir, 1967; Howell and Morford, 1961; Howell and Morford, 1964; Morgan and Adamson, 1959; Sorani, 1966.

YOU SHOULD REMEMBER THAT:

Calisthenic and weight training programs, when they are *not* supplemented with CR conditioning, are not adequate to develop general physical fitness because they fail to improve CR capacity to any significant degree.

CR fitness is probably the most important quality of physical fitness and should not be neglected or excluded for other advantages such as physique, strength, and so on.

Circuit training provides for individual goals, self-testing, and competition with self or others. It combines CR conditioning with other needs, self-prescribed and highly personalized.

One Step
Further

7

HISTORICAL, CULTURAL
AND
PHILOSOPHICAL ASPECTS

The purpose of this chapter is to help you:
1. Develop some understanding of the history of training
and physical fitness programs, and their influence
on our culture and vice versa
2. Appreciate some of the philosophical
aspects of training and physical fitness

THE HISTORY OF TRAINING

The cave man probably participated in no programs of conditioning, training, or general physical fitness unless one considers a way of life a conditioning and training program. Strength, endurance, and physical skills were not qualities about which the cave man debated. Without these qualities survival was only a remote possibility. There are no records (nor is there any logic) to indicate that prehistoric man engaged in any systematic form of training, conditioning, or physical activity. Physical activity was his life.

The earliest recorded attempt at a systematized program for the improvement of health and physical fitness may have been a form of medical gymnastics called Cong Fou, practiced by the ancient Chinese (about 2700 B.C.). This program combined stretching and breathing exercises and was usually performed in the kneeling or sitting position.

Archeological findings provide us with evidence that ancient Egyptians (around 2000 B.C.) participated in boxing, wrestling, and other athletic events. It is logical to assume that those participating in such activities prepared for these events with some kind of conditioning and training program. We do know that in preparation for the Olympic Games (probably initiated sometime before 776 B.C.) Greek competitors spent at least 10 months in hard training and conditioning exercises. Though their viewpoints on physical conditioning differed (from the Spartan philosophy of training for military purposes to the Athenian belief that beauty and the harmony of mind and body were as important as the military training aspects), the Greeks nevertheless produced systematic approaches to the improvement of physical qualities and skills. Plato certainly believed in the harmony of body and spirit but he also believed that excessive attention to development of the body was undesirable. He believed that the man who "takes violent exercise and is a great feeder becomes filled with pride at the high condition of his body, but if he does nothing else he becomes fierce, ignorant and dull," like a wild beast (Jowett, 1928).

Galen (131-201 A.D.), appears to have been the first "team physician" in history. Some of his viewpoints are extremely interesting historically (Green, 1958). He claimed that exercise improved strength by hardening the organs, increasing respiration and intrinsic warmth, in turn producing a better nutritional state of the body, and improved metabolism and elimination. He recommended exercising before meals to improve digestion and suggested that those who were training for health alone should practice moderation in their exercise, massage, bathing, food, and sleep. He suggested that they should stop exercise before they became fatigued, but stated that in training for competition "It is necessary for athletes, in order that they may prepare themselves for their labors in competitions, to practice immoderately sometimes all day at their objective exercise, which they call training" (Green, 1958). It is apparent that by this time in history man had become sufficiently relieved of the constant necessity of being vigorously active that he required special conditioning and training programs in order to maintain enough strength and endurance to participate in vigorous activity.

Rome was characterized by its spectacles, requiring no citizen participation (Van Daten, Mitchell, and Bennett, 1953). There is no evidence that the average citizen participated in any kind of improvement programs, at least physically speaking. The soldiers trained for battle and the gladiators did train, of course, for their special kind of spectacular brutality. It has been reported that the gladiators believed strongly in the value of massage after exercise to loosen the tightened muscles.

In more modern times, the Swedes and Germans popularized formal gymnastics and formalized calisthenics for the improvement of physical fitness; the English emphasized the value of games and sports, not so much in contributing to physical fitness as in developing desirable social qualities. The colonial period in our own country was characterized by an agrarian existence, which required hard physical work and no additional effort at improving physical fitness.

The draft rejection statistics during World War I caused some concern and discussion about the state of health and physical fitness in the United States and, apparently, even greater concern during World War II. But nothing formal was proposed as a solution until President Dwight D. Eisenhower established the President's Council on Youth Fitness in 1956. This motivated a renewed emphasis on the value of physical fitness among our youth. But it was not until President John F. Kennedy changed the name and the emphasis of this President's Council in 1961 that significant emphasis was placed upon physical fitness for the entire population. The President's Council on Physical Fitness began to promote adult as well as youth fitness. Since then there has been a deluge of printed matter and exercise gimmicks aimed at improvement of physical fitness.

THE PRESENT

It is difficult to say whether Americans, on the whole, are more physically fit than they were 10 years ago, but without hesitation we can say that physical fitness levels could still afford to be improved.

There is little question that physical fitness and conditioning are a part of our culture. One needs only to peruse the popular literature of the past 5 to 10 years to see that the public (or at least the publishers, who seem to have an ear for the wants and needs of the public) is aware of and at least intellectually interested in matters concerning health and physical fitness. Much has been written about the detrimental effects of automation and an overmechanized society on the physical fitness and mental alertness of our people. Alarmists have pointed to the historical fact that 19 of the world's 21 great civilizations crumbled when their people gradually changed from a mentally and physically active existence to a physically sedentary and morally stagnant way of life (Toynbee, 1946). It has been estimated that on the average we spend only about 1 hour in physical participation for every 75 hours as spectators viewing movies, television, sporting events, and so on. It remains to be seen whether the written word, federal, state, and local programs, or man's own informed self-analysis will in any way appreciably improve the average state of physical fitness in our country.

There is another aspect of physical fitness, culturally speaking, which may be a problem worth attacking. The very real difference between "athletic competition" and "health and physical fitness" is not apparent to the majority of our population. Parents do not encourage their youngsters to participate (nor do the youngsters themselves participate) in Little League sports to improve their health and physical fitness but, rather, to compete and, hopefully, to succeed at competition. Whereas there may be nothing wrong with this attitude, to promote such competition as aiding health and physical fitness may be misleading. For example, Little League baseball affords very little of the kind of exercise that actually improves circulo-respiratory fitness, strength, muscular endurance, and flexibility. It is unfortunate that culturally we accept athletic and sports competition as synonymous with health and physical fitness. There may or may not be a correspondence, depending on the activity.

One final cultural consideration bears mentioning. In far too many localities, women and girls, when they have reached a so-called "feminine age," about the time of puberty, are supposed to act in a "ladylike fashion," participating in only a minimum of physical activity. Space does not permit us to discuss this problem fully; suffice it to say that normal girls and women need physical activity just as much as men do. Furthermore, participation in reasonably vigorous activity of a generalized nature will not produce any physical or psychological changes that will make a woman appear or act masculine. The atypical, "masculine" woman sports champion was that way before she became a champion and did not change as a result of her sports participation!

Regardless of personal convictions, it is certainly clear that one's physical activity or his inactivity is intimately bound up in his philosophy of life and goals. Some feel that keeping healthy and physically fit is as much religious as it is personal. On the other hand, some believe that it is best to "live fast, die young, and have a beautiful corpse." Both of these extreme viewpoints obviously reflect one's philosophy of life and his view of his role in society. It is impossible to separate mind and body, and the state of one's body does affect his mental processes; one's philosophy depends on those mental processes. Physical activity, whether directly or indirectly, does affect and is affected by one's philosophy of life.

THE HISTORY OF TRAINING AND PHYSICAL FITNESS PROGRAMS SHOWS THAT:

Man has not always needed special activity programs to maintain health and fitness. At one time, physical activity *was* his life.

Man's civilized state has created for many people a need for nonoccupational, supplementary physical activity. Thus, we have training, physical fitness, and conditioning programs.

Physical fitness and training intimately affect and are affected by our culture.

One's personal philosophy of life often reflects his view of the role of physical activity in his life.

8

BENEFITS AND LIMITATIONS OF FITNESS, TRAINING, AND CONDITIONING

The purpose of this chapter is to help you understand:
1. *The physiological benefits of physical activity, and its limitations*
2. *The psychological benefits of physical activity, and its limitations*
3. *The social benefits of physical activity, and its limitations*

If you are to be knowledgeable about conditioning, training, and physical fitness you will need to know what will and what will not happen as a result of these various programs. You will want to know what the real benefits of general physical fitness are, and to know the benefits and the extent of these benefits for each quality that contributes to general physical fitness. It is quite obvious that any specific training program that is intended to improve some measurable performance either does or does not succeed. But it is *not* so obvious what other benefits occur as a result of conditioning, training, or physical fitness programs. The evidence (as well as lack of evidence) is presented here in summarized form; if you wish to delve more deeply into any aspect of this summary, you will find the references most useful.

Benefits and limitations will be discussed under the three general headings *physiological*, *psychological*, and *social*.

PHYSIOLOGICAL BENEFITS OF PHYSICAL ACTIVITY AND ITS LIMITATIONS

Specific Benefits of Improved Circulo-Respiratory Fitness

There is evidence to suggest at least four benefits of improved CR capacity. It should be obvious that the amount of benefit depends on the level of CR fitness.

1. The most obvious benefit of improved CR fitness is improved circulo-respiratory work capacity (Johnson et al., 1966; Moncrieff, 1963). Simply stated, the person with a high level of CR fitness is able to endure in activities that are limited by the ability of the heart and lungs to continue functioning efficiently and without intolerable discomfort. To be sure, there is a high degree of specificity involved. The individual whose CR capacity has been improved via a swimming program can swim longer than can one conditioned via a running program, but he would fare poorly in comparison to the runner in a test of running endurance. Nevertheless, there is some transfer, so that either of these persons would normally be able to outlast an extremely sedentary person in either running or swimming.

2. A second benefit is preparedness for emergencies (Yost, 1967) which require a strong and efficient circulo-respiratory system. Where persistence in a generalized, strenuous activity is essential to the safety and well-being of self or others, the person with the strong circulo-respiratory system is at an obvious advantage.

3. There is some evidence that improvement in CR fitness provides a concomitant increase in the efficiency of daily living (Johnson et al., 1966). The person with CR fitness should be able to carry out his daily activities and routine more efficiently, with less fatigue, and with greater reserve, so that his activities toward the end of his work day are as efficient and nonfatiguing as they were at the start of the day. This benefit, however, has not been completely substantiated through measurement.

4. There is strong evidence, although most of it is indirect, that the active individual is less likely to suffer from *coronary heart disease* than is the very sedentary person (Brunner and Manelis, 1960; Hedley, 1939; Morris and Crawford, 1958; Morris et al., 1953; Pedley, 1942; Ryle and Russel, 1949; Taylor, 1960; Zukel, 1959) (see Fig. 8-1). He is also less likely to have a severe and fatal heart attack if he does have one (Brunner and Manelis, 1960). He is not as likely to suffer from coronary heart disease as early in life as is the sedentary person. In some instances the indirect evidence does not specifi-

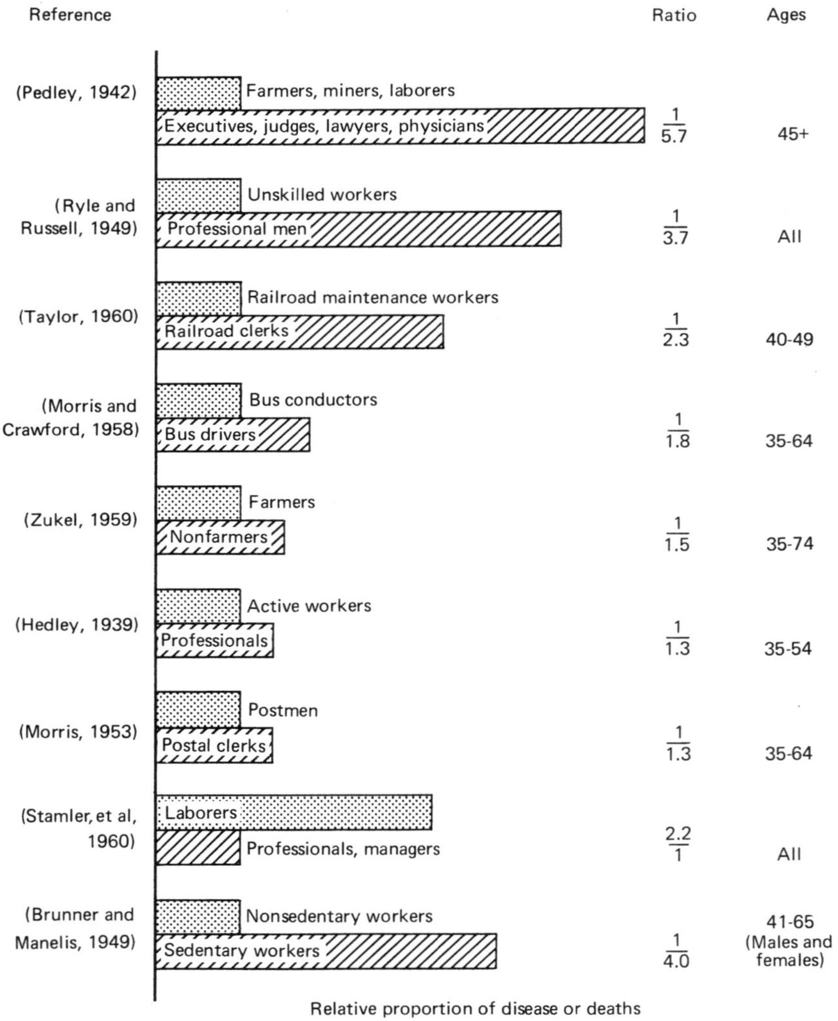

FIGURE 8-1. Summary of studies comparing active and inactive occupations with respect to coronary heart disease or death due to coronary disease

cally relate to CR fitness, but rather to physical activity in general. Nevertheless, all of the evidence taken together logically points to CR fitness as the key component of general physical fitness in prevention and delay of coronary heart disease. It is important to keep in mind that the evidence is *not* direct that a high level of CR fitness will provide *immunity* against atherosclerosis and coronary heart disease. Nevertheless, regular physical activity, especially that which improves the CR capacity, is a sensible and scientifically sound measure that considerably improves the odds against your suffering from degenerative disease of the circulatory system and heart.

It is not only the lack of direct evidence that motivates us to caution against the assumption that CR fitness provides certain immunity against coronary heart disease. One must also bear in mind that factors other than lack of physical exercise have been identified as possible contributors to coronary heart disease and atherosclerosis (Johnson et al., 1966). These are: (1) excess body fat; (2) anxiety, stress, and tension; (3) excess intake of fat and simple sugar; (4) cigarette smoking; and (5) heredity.

Muscular Endurance

The most obvious benefit of improved muscular endurance is the ability to persist for longer periods of time in physical tasks using specific muscle groups. Again the principle of specificity is important: Running, for example, will not increase appreciably the muscular endurance required for repeated forceful arm and shoulder movements. A concomitant benefit, of course, is preparedness for emergencies that might require long-term and repeated application of muscular force.

Strength

Needless to say, there are emergency situations in which greater strength may be a distinct advantage. A less obvious benefit of adequate muscular strength relates to general health. We refer to the little-known relationship between the strength of the abdominal muscles and the flexibility of the hamstring muscles of the legs in controlling the tilt of the pelvis (Flint, 1968; Kraus and Raab, 1961). The tilt of the pelvis, in turn, affects the curvature in the lower back region which, when it becomes exaggerated, can lead to excessive tension in the area and to what is commonly referred to as "low back pain." It has been estimated that some 80 percent of those who suffer low back pain suffer because of a muscular rather than a functional disorder. We are not implying that abdominal strength and hamstring flexibility automatically prevent all lower back disorders, but these specific aspects of physical fitness will tend to lessen the probability that low back pain will occur.

Flexibility

In addition to the role that hamstring flexibility can play in prevention of low back pain, greater flexibility of a joint should reduce the chances for muscle stress and injuries that result from overstretching. It is obvious that no amount of flexibility can prevent injury when the muscle's ability to stretch has been exceeded, but that point will not be reached as soon when flexibility has been increased. In highly specialized kinds of work (and especially in certain of the performing arts and in tumbling and apparatus competition), flexibility is a prerequisite to success.

General Physical Fitness

The three most common and most important questions relating to the benefits of physical fitness are: (1) Does physical fitness increase length of life? (2) Does physical fitness prevent or reduce chances of disease and infection? and (3) Does general physical fitness contribute to sports success?

Fitness and longevity. Although there is no direct experimental evidence that the physically fit person tends to live longer, excluding of course deaths from accident and suicide, indirect evidence and logic support a rather modest claim that the physically fit person, all other things being equal, may expect to live at least slightly longer than his sedentary and unfit counterpart. Hammond's study (1964) of over one million persons (see Fig. 8-2) and evidence that strongly suggests that more active persons suffer fewer heart attacks and less severe ones (see page 83), provides the theoretical basis for the position that the physically fit person improves his chances of a long life. Unfortunately, longevity studies have been based primarily on college letter-winners versus non-letter-winners (Montoye et al., 1957; Montoye, 1960), and they have not taken into account in any way the amount of activity engaged in by the individuals after they left college. Although direct and conclusive evidence is lacking to support either a claim that the physically fit live longer or that they die sooner, there is sufficient justification to adopt the position that the physically fit person should live longer, all other things being equal.

Resistance to infection and disease. Many kinds of claims for the value of physical fitness have been made. Perhaps the most ridiculous, at least in terms of what scientists now know, is the claim that physical fitness will prevent

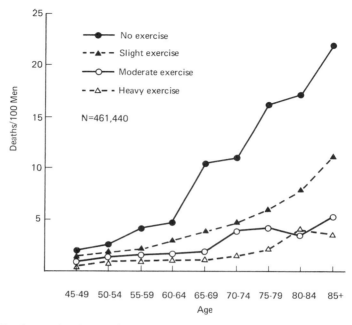

FIGURE 8-2. Death rate by degree of regular exercise and age group during a period of one year (data from Hammond, 1964)

cancer. It is equally foolish to claim that physical fitness prevents infectious disease. In fact, there is some evidence that fatiguing exercise may hasten the onset of certain infectious diseases if a person has been exposed to the disease-causing organism (Johnson et al., 1966). On the other hand, if we assume that fatigue hastens or increases the chances for infection from the invading organism, then the physically fit person might theoretically prevent infection if his fitness level keeps him from reaching the state of fatigue or exhaustion. Although this relationship is highly theoretical, there is some work that supports it (Merrill and Howe, 1928; Zimkin, 1961).

Physical fitness and sports success. Some coaches, physical educators, and physiologists argue that general physical fitness is necessary for championship or even moderately successful sports performance; others feel that fitness is not essential to excellent performance in certain sports activities. They give examples of championship athletes who, although they are well conditioned and trained in the particular movement or activity necessary for participation, have a very low level of general physical fitness, especially of

CR capacity. In all honesty, we do not know the answer. It is certain that one needs to develop at least the kind of endurance necessary for him to complete his event again and again as many times as required in the most lengthy competition. Perhaps this kind of specific endurance is more important than circulo-respiratory endurance, but it may also be that improved CR endurance aids in improving endurance in the specific activity or movement. An example might be jumping and rebounding abilities in basketball. A man who can jump 2½' from the floor in the first 5 minutes of the game but who cannot jump more than 2' at the end of the game is not fit for his sport. But whether CR fitness in excess of that required to run up and down the floor and make the necessary offensive and defensive movements for 40 minutes would aid in improving that jumping endurance is problematical. Certainly, repeated jumping, with the attempt to attain maximal height on each jump, would help to improve jumping endurance.

Certainly in a sport or activity that requires CR fitness, performance should be improved by increasing this kind of fitness; and in a sport that requires any of the aspects of general physical fitness, improved general fitness should improve performance of the sport.

PSYCHOLOGICAL BENEFITS OF PHYSICAL ACTIVITY AND ITS LIMITATIONS

The science of psychology has advanced rapidly in recent years and certain aspects of man's psychological behavior have become at least somewhat easier to assess. Nevertheless, claims for the psychological benefits of physical activity, by nature of the difficulty in measuring objectively what is termed "psychological behavior," are difficult to support. We feel intuitively that regular physical activity can have certain psychological benefits for some individuals under certain circumstances.

There is some evidence that tends to support intuition. This evidence will be noted where applicable, but for the most part, the following discussion will be based upon observation, experience with others, personal experience, and intuition.

The most positive statement that would still be intellectually honest is that physical fitness or the specific activities involved in its achievement and maintenance may have a positive effect on the following psychological characteristics of some individuals (Cowell, 1960):

1. sense of well-being
2. positive mental health and the prevention of emotional illness
3. relaxation and release of tensions and anxieties

4. personality and attitudes
5. mental alertness, learning capacity, and mental efficiency
6. sensory and perceptual awareness and responsiveness
7. positive self-image
8. mental rehabilitation

Whether or not a positive effect occurs is entirely dependent upon the specific interaction for an individual among his psyche, the environment, and the particular activity.

There seems to be considerable overlapping and interaction among the benefits listed. For example, one's self-image would certainly interact with the particular activity and the environment and, in conjunction with one's personality, determine whether or not relaxation occurred as a result of the activity. You can see how someone with a poor self-image might become less relaxed after a poor round of golf, whereas a person with a strong self-image, under exactly the same conditions, might be thoroughly relaxed because he attributed his poor game that day to something other than his own shortcomings. In any event certain psychological benefits can be derived from physical activity but we should like to emphasize the word *can* and to further emphasize the concept that changes in behavior resulting from physical activity, like anything else which can cause changes in behavior and attitude, are entirely an individual matter.

SOCIAL BENEFITS OF PHYSICAL ACTIVITY AND ITS LIMITATIONS

It is difficult if not impossible to separate social development from psychological development. However, in considering social benefits, we will limit ourselves to those kinds of changes that relate to one's ability to be an effective participant in society.

The important question is what, if any, contributions to the process through which you learn to be a participant in society can you expect from your participation in conditioning, training, or physical fitness activities? First, since it is generally accepted that most people are by nature gregarious, if you choose activities that involve other persons you are providing for yourself an opportunity to meet the need for social interaction. Second, you should keep clearly in mind that it is not the activity itself that is responsible for social development but, rather, the circumstances associated with it (Cratty, 1967). Third, you should understand that social development related to one particular role (for example, tennis player) does not necessarily carry over to other roles (Kenyon, 1968). If social development is poor, this lack of transfer may be desirable (for example, poor social development on the golf course or tennis court does not necessarily carry over into one's daily interpersonal relationships). Finally, it is important to recognize that an audience, be it one other person or a large group of participants, does have a varying effect, depending on the individual, on one's response in any given social setting (Cratty, 1967). This holds true for participation in physical activities as well as in other social settings.

As with psychological benefits, the activities included in conditioning, training, and physical fitness *may* contribute to social development, but such development is entirely dependent upon the interaction of the individual's personality, the environmental setting, and the activity itself, including when and how often it is performed. Something that is experienced only once may have a profound effect upon one person's social development and not another's. It should be clear that physical activity is *not* the solution to all of our social problems. But it can and often does contribute to social development and there is evidence to support the claim with respect to the following specific kinds of social development. In summary (Cowell, 1960; Cratty, 1967; Kenyon, 1968), there is evidence that athletic ability and sports participation, physical skill, strength, physique and body size, vitality, and positive health can have a positive effect on: (1) social adjustment, (2) popularity, (3) social prestige and status, and (4) leadership. It is important to keep in mind that physical activity experiences can result in *negative* social development; the same game that provides *positive* social development for one individual who is successful may provide for the unsuccessful person in the same game some kind of negative social development. In short, you may or may not derive social benefits from physical activities; whether or not you do is entirely an individual matter.

YOU SHOULD NOW BE AWARE THAT:

Physiological benefits can result from physical fitness improvement.

Such benefits can be classed as health-related, related to preparation for emergency, and related to improved sports performance.

Psychological and social benefits can also result from physical activity programs.

Benefits derived from physical fitness programs are individual, and negative as well as positive changes may occur.

9

APPLICABLE PRINCIPLES
OF MOTOR LEARNING

The purpose of this chapter is to help you:
1. Become aware of the principles of motor learning
2. Be able to apply these principles
to conditioning and training programs

Motor-learning principles are considerably more applicable to what we have called *training* (leading to externally measurable performance) than to conditioning or to the attainment of physical fitness. There are principles of conditioning and physical fitness attainment, but those principles do not relate so much to motor performance.

There is still a great deal to be learned about the principles of motor learning; most of the ones that have been isolated by experimental research cannot be stated as laws. Nevertheless, there are certain general principles that may aid you considerably in setting up and carrying out a program to improve any quality of motor ability.

1. Improvement in certain aspects of motor ability may be limited by inadequate levels of general physical fitness or by the lack of some specific quality of physical fitness (Singer, 1968).

2. The individual's emotional state may have a significant effect (either positive or negative) upon his ability to improve a motor skill (Singer, 1968).

3. Adequate motivation is almost essential for motor learning to occur (Singer, 1968).

4. Practice does not automatically insure improvement in a motor skill; you may regress if you practice incorrectly (Singer, 1968).

5. Motor learning may be negatively affected by continuing to practice a skill after neuromuscular "fatigue" has set in (Seyffarth, 1940). Keep in mind that this kind of impairment of the functional capacity of the neuromuscular system (commonly called fatigue) may be very subtle and is not necessarily associated with what one might call "all-out fatigue" as exemplified by fatigue from distance running or swimming.

6. In general, when a motor skill involves speed and accuracy, it is best to work at improving both at the same time; in complicated skills where it is impossible to achieve both simultaneously, speed should probably be reduced until a reasonable degree of accuracy can be attained (Johnson et al., 1966).

7. In general, it is preferable to practice the entire skill in a total and integrated fashion, rather than to break it down into component parts and then try to put the parts together. People vary in their capacity to learn a skill by the "whole method," and some persons learn some skills best by breaking them down into two or more component parts (Johnson et al., 1966).

8. Although mental practice cannot replace actual practice, it is possible that mentally rehearsing the skill may provide a basis for or actually contribute to faster learning of a skill (Johnson et al., 1966).

9. In general, it is better to practice a skill more often for shorter periods of time than to mass all practice into few practice sessions (Singer, 1968).

10. In skills that involve rapid repetition of movement, so that the joint or joints are alternately flexing and extending, it is possible that "extra" effort can be so extreme that the muscles of extension and flexion may actually be working against each other and thus impair rather than improve performance (Johnson et al., 1966).

11. There is, in general, great specificity in motor learning, and learning of one skill does not automatically transfer to learning of another skill. There is some generality and some transfer can occur, but only when the movements are very similar in nature (Singer, 1968).

(Many of these principles are referred to in the general principles relating to improvement of specific motor abilities, Chapter 5.)

AFTER READING THIS CHAPTER, YOU SHOULD KNOW THAT:

A poor emotional state, fatigue, incorrect practice, or trying too hard may be detrimental to motor learning.

Adequate fitness levels, proper motivation, mental rehearsal of the task, and frequent short practice sessions may aid motor learning.

10

WHY IMPROVEMENT OCCURS

The purpose of this chapter is to help you understand
the theoretical mechanisms behind the improvement of:
1. Circulo-respiratory fitness
2. Muscular strength
3. Muscular endurance
4. Flexibility
5. Motor ability

If you are the kind of person who often asks the question "why?," if you are intrigued by the possibility of learning more about changes in behavior and performance, or if you are or would like to be a student of physical fitness and its associated training and conditioning phenomena, this section should provide you with some useful basic information. It will also draw your attention to references that will provide you with a greater depth of understanding about conditioning and training. A knowledge of the mechanisms involved in improvement may also provide you with greater insight into the programs that can best contribute to your improvement.

The established mechanisms of improvement of the various qualities of physical fitness and motor ability will be presented in summarized form, along with those that are presently theoretical. You may refer to the bibliography for further detailed information. Any statement followed by a **T** is one which, to our knowledge, is logical and tenable, but is not supported by adequate experimental evidence.

IMPROVEMENT IN CIRCULO-RESPIRATORY FITNESS (WORK CAPACITY)

The ability to persist for longer periods of time in reasonably strenuous large-muscle activities as a result of conditioning is probably the result of several if not all of the following changes in physiological function. It should be quite obvious that the magnitude of the improvement in work capacity and, thus, the changes in physiological functions, are dependent upon the nature, intensity, regularity, and duration of a given conditioning program. At any rate, nearly all of the following changes do occur as a result of regular participation in programs that place demands upon the circulatory and respiratory systems.

1. Decreased resting and exercise heart rate (Henry, 1954; Johnson, 1965; Knehr, Dill, and Newfeld, 1942) (see Fig. 10-1).

2. Increased stroke volume and cardiac output during exercise (Chapman and Mitchell, 1965). (That is, the conditioned heart almost invariably ejects more blood per beat and circulates more blood to the body per minute than does the nonconditioned heart.)

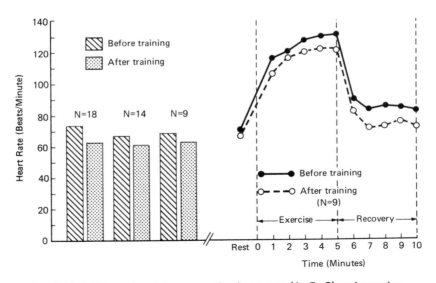

FIGURE 10-1. Effect of training on resting heart rate (A, B, C) and exercise-recovery heart rate (D) (data from F. Henry, 1954; Knehr, 1942; Johnson, Updyke, and W. Henry, 1965)

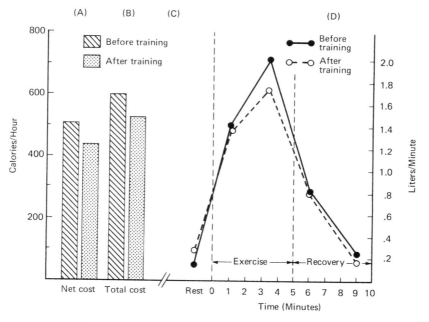

FIGURE 10-2. Effect of training on exercise energy cost and on oxygen utilization during exercise (based on Johnson, Updyke, and F. Henry, 1965)

3. There may be an increase in total blood volume and in blood hemoglobin (Kjellberg, Rudhe, and Sjostrand). (That is, oxygen-carrying capacity of the blood may increase, which means that more oxygen is available to the tissues.)

4. There may be an increased maximal O_2 utilization (Balke and Clarke). (That is, the tissues of the body may become capable of utilizing more oxygen per minute.)

5. There is usually a decreased oxygen requirement, at least for a specific and given task (Johnson, Updyke, and Henry, 1965). (That is, reduced utilization of fuel may provide for greater endurance) (see Fig. 10-2).

6. There may be an increased O_2 debt tolerance (Karpovich, 1965; Morehouse and Miller, 1963; Taylor, 1960).

7. There may be an increase in the vital capacity of the lungs and in the maximal breathing capacity (Bachman and Horvath, 1968; Cureton, 1951). (That is, ability to move more air into and out of the lungs per minute makes

it possible to provide more oxygen to the blood and to remove carbon dioxide from the blood faster.)

8. The heart muscle itself may undergo hypertrophy (Steinhaus, 1963). (That is, the muscle itself may become larger and stronger.) The heart muscle may develop an improved blood supply through an increase in or an opening up of capillaries supplying the heart muscle (Steinhaus, 1963).

9. The heart muscle may become more efficient (Mallerowicz, 1960). (That is, it may accomplish more work with less oxygen demand.)

IMPROVEMENT IN MUSCULAR STRENGTH

The most obvious mechanism for increased muscular strength is hypertrophy or increase in size of the muscle fibers and, in turn, an increase in the size of the muscle itself. It has been well established that the muscle fiber exerts its contractile force roughly in proportion to its cross-sectional area (Karpovich, 1965). That is, the larger the muscle fiber, the greater the contractile force it can exert when stimulated. But muscle hypertrophy cannot possibly explain the apparent increase in muscular strength that can occur in a period of one or two days. Since it is illogical to assume that significant muscle hypertrophy occurs in 24 hours, when one lifts 75 pounds one day and then is able to lift 90 pounds the following day, some explanation other than hypertrophy is necessary. There are at least three other plausible explanations for some increase in muscular strength. Probably these occur concomitantly with hypertrophy so that increases in strength are greater than those which could be accounted for by hypertrophy alone.

Studies have provided some evidence that the *inhibition-facilitation ratio* of the central nervous system can be changed to improve strength (Johnson et al., 1966). It has been claimed that if it were not for the inhibitory impulses of the central nervous system, muscles could be contracted so forcefully that they would be literally torn away from their attachments to the bones. Thus, if these inhibitory impulses can be reduced somewhat and facilitory (or positive) impulses increased, greater application of force can result.

There is evidence that as one develops and perfects any skilled movement, even one as apparently simple as flexing the elbow, coordination of the motor units of the various muscles involved in the movement improves. As skill in a movement increases, the same motor units are always active and always in the same sequence (Seyffarth, 1940). Thus it appears that the neuromuscular system is capable of causing improvement in its own efficiency so that application of force may be increased.

The connective tissue that supports and provides a framework for the muscle may be strengthened and toughened as a result of conditioning (Steinhaus, 1963). This may also provide some strength increment over and above that which occurs via the mechanisms already mentioned (**T**).

IMPROVEMENT IN MUSCULAR ENDURANCE

To date, the most plausible hypothetical mechanisms contributing to improved muscular endurance are: (1) increased capillarization in the muscles, (2) a change in the inhibition-facilitation ratio, and (3) increased neuromuscular coordination. All of these theoretical mechanisms are supported by some experimental evidence, but there is insufficient evidence to allow any firm conclusions.

Increased capillarization in specific muscles as a result of regular exercise was demonstrated experimentally some time ago (see Steinhaus, 1963). Unfortunately, there has been no systematic follow-up. Nevertheless, the hypothesis that increased blood supply is at least partly responsible for increased muscular endurance is a tenable one (**T**). Experimental studies involving hypnosis have provided some evidence that reduction in inhibition, increase in facilitation, or both, may be responsible for dramatic increases in muscular endurance (Johnson and Kramer, 1961). Though these increases certainly occur, attributing such increases to a change in the inhibition-facilitation ratio is more a matter of scientific logic than it is physiological fact (**T**). With respect to improved coordination within the neuromuscular system (Seyffarth, 1940), the same evidence that leads us to suspect that this phenomenon may be partly responsible for increases in muscular strength leads us to conclude that such a change may also account for some of the improvement in muscular endurance (**T**).

IMPROVEMENT IN FLEXIBILITY

Very little is known about the physiological changes involved in improvement in flexibility. It is obvious, however, that such changes can and do occur and that they somehow relate to an increased ability of the structural elements of the total muscle to be stretched without pain or damage. It is also important to note that a muscle can be increased in strength and that the increase in strength need not be associated with a concomitant decrease in the flexibility of the joint affected, provided, of course, that regular stretching exercises are included along with the weight training exercises.

IMPROVEMENT IN MOTOR ABILITY

The mechanisms involved in improvement of the various qualities of motor ability are not well established. It seems reasonable to assume, however, that the improvement results from improved coordination within the nervous system itself (Seyffarth, 1940) (**T**). There is some evidence that the transmission of nervous impulses involved in a given skilled movement is improved and facilitated by repetition. It also seems reasonable that certain kinds of motor abilities may be improved where improved strength, flexibility, or muscular endurance would contribute directly to improvement. (**T**). For instance, assuming time of force application is not changed, increased strength (greater force applied) should increase power.

KEEP IN MIND THAT:

An understanding of how improvement occurs can aid one in planning his program, especially in keeping with the principles of *demand* and *specificity*.

There are research-substantiated explanations (in addition to theoretical explanations) for the improvement of fitness qualities.

There is less evidence upon which to base explanations for motor ability improvement than there is for other types of improvement.

11

NUTRITIONAL AND DIETARY CONSIDERATIONS

The purpose of this chapter is to help you
understand and be able to use the basic principles
of nutrition and diet as they apply to:
1. Health
2. Physical fitness
3. Performance

Although a great deal has been written (and thousands of people have *believed* what has been written) about various health foods and their beneficial effects upon health, physical fitness, and performance, experimental evidence has failed to lend significant support to any of the health food fads. To date, the following principles of nutrition as related to physical fitness, training, and conditioning seem to be scientifically valid:

1. A normal, well-balanced diet, increased when necessary to meet the requirements of increased physical activity, will not be improved by more or additional kinds of nutrients. Additional nutrients will not contribute to improved fitness or performance (Mayer and Bullen, 1960). The normal, well-balanced diet (Fig. 11-1) to which we refer includes the following:

   a. At least 1 gram of *protein* per day per kilogram of body weight (that is, about ½ gram per day per pound of body weight).

   b. From 20 to 25 percent of the total Calories from fats ("Present Knowledge of Fat," 1966) about two-thirds of

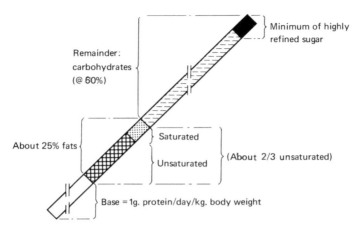

Minimum of highly
refined sugar

Remainder:
carbohydrates
(@ 60%)

About 25% fats

Saturated

Unsaturated

(About 2/3 unsaturated)

Base = 1g. protein/day/kg. body weight

FIGURE 11-1. Components of a normal balanced diet

which are consumed in the form of *unsaturated fats* (soft fats and oils). Fats should not be eliminated from the diet but they should not be consumed in excess of 25 percent of the total caloric intake and the majority should be of the unsaturated variety. Excessive fat intake and especially excessive saturated fat intake have been linked to high cholesterol levels, atherosclerosis, and coronary heart disease. Nevertheless, some fat intake is essential to proper nourishment of the body's cells.

c. The remainder (roughly 60 percent) of the caloric intake should be in the form of carbohydrates. There is evidence that a minimum (no more than 90 grams per day) of the carbohydrate intake should be in the form of highly purified sugars such as table sugar, pastries and cakes, soft drinks, and fruits ("Present Knowledge of Carbohydrates," 1966; Yudkin, 1964; Yudkin and Morland, 1967). The majority should be in the form of starches. The evidence on excessive simple sugar intake points to its correlation with increased likelihood of atherosclerosis and coronary heart disease (Yudkin, 1964; Yudkin and Morland, 1967).

d. Adequate vitamin, mineral, and water intake is equally essential to a diet of sufficient calories and properly balanced with respect to fats, proteins, and carbohydrates provides adequate vitamins and minerals, and most people can rely on their thirst mechanism to tell them the amount of water and liquid intake essential for good health.

2. Glucose as a fuel requires less oxygen per unit of energy expended than

do fats. There is some evidence that performance, especially of an endurance nature, may benefit from a slight increase in the carbohydrate intake (Mayer and Bullen, 1960). This increase should not be at the expense of protein and should not be carried to extremes.

3. During normal growth periods and when one is attempting to increase muscle mass, protein intake may need to be increased above the minimum daily requirement recommended above (Mayer and Bullen, 1960).

4. Vitamin, mineral, and hormone supplements have not been proven to benefit performance or general physical fitness unless the individual has a particular deficiency which is met by a therapeutic level of supplementation.

We do not yet have enough scientific evidence to explain all the principles and mechanisms behind training, conditioning, and physical fitness. Nevertheless, specially designed and regularly practiced exercise programs, hand in hand with proper diet and mental attitude, can lead to improvement of general fitness and aspects of physical performance.

AFTER READING THIS CHAPTER, YOU SHOULD REALIZE THAT:

The best diet for a person in training is essentially the same as would be recommended for a normal individual.

A good diet for such a person should provide for growth if he is still growing, for increase in muscle mass if desired, and for adequate energy.

An inadequate diet can hamper performance.

APPENDIX A

Rating of Sports and Activities for Developing Fitness and Motor Ability

3-High value; 2-Medium value; 1-Low value; (0)-Doubtful value; 0-No value (All activities rated 1, 2, 3 vary in value, depending upon regularity, intensity, and/or duration of exercise.) (Recommended age is dependent upon physical fitness and health of individual.) C = Coordination; P = Power; A = Agility; B = Balance.

ACTIVITY	CR CAPACITY	MUSCULAR ENDURANCE	STRENGTH	FLEXIBILITY	OTHER	AGE RANGE RECOMMENDED
Archery	0	3	1.5	(0)		All ages
Badminton (singles)	2.5	1.5	0	(0)	A,C	Under 50
Badminton (doubles)	1	1.5	0	(0)	A,C	Under 60
Basketball	2.5	2.5	(0)	(0)	A,C,P,B	Under 30
Baseball	1	2	(0)	(0)	C,P,B	Under 45
Bicycling (recreation)	2.5	3	1.5	(0)		All ages
Bowling	0	1	0	0	C,B	All ages
Calisthenics	1.5-3.0	2-3	1	1-3	C,B	All ages
Canoeing, Rowing (recreation)	2-3	2-3	1-2	(0)	C	All ages
(competitive)	3	3	2-3	(0)	C	Under 30
Field Hockey	3	2-3	1	(0)	C,B,A	Under 30
Football	1.5	2-3	1-2	(0)	C,A,P	Under 30
Golf	1-2	(0)	0	(0)	C,P	All ages
Handball (singles)	2.5	1.5	0	(0)	C,P,B,A	Under 45

ACTIVITY	CR CAPACITY	MUSCULAR ENDURANCE	STRENGTH	FLEXIBILITY	OTHER	AGE RANGE RECOMMENDED
Handball (doubles)	1	1.5	0	(0)	C,P,B,A	Under 60
Apparatus	0	2-3	2.5	1-2	C,B,A	Under 45
Tumbling	0	2	1.5	2-3	C,B,A	Under 50
Hiking	2	2	(0)	(0)		All ages
Skating, speed	2.5-3	2-3	1	(0)	C,B,A	Under 45
Skiing	1-3	1-3	1-2	1	C,B,A	Under 45
Soccer	3	2-3	1	(0)	C,P,A	Under 45
Softball	1	1-2	(0)	(0)	C,P,A	Under 50
Swimming (recreation)	1-3	1-3	1	(0)		All ages
(competitive)	2-3	1-3	2	1-2		Under 30
Tennis, singles	2.5	1.5	(0)	(0)	C,P,A,B	Under 45
Tennis, doubles	1	1.5	(0)	(0)	C,P,A,B	Under 50
Jogging	2-3	2-3	(0)	(0)		All ages
Running	3	2-3	(0)	(0)		Under 45
Rope Skipping	2-3	2-3	(0)	(0)	C,B	Under 40
Volleyball	(0)	1-2	(0)	(0)	C,B,P,A	All ages
Wrestling	2-3	2-3	1-2	2-3	C,B,P,A	Under 30

APPENDIX B

Desirable Weights for Men of Ages 25 and Over: Weight in Pounds According to Frame (in Indoor Clothing)

HEIGHT (WITH SHOES ON— 1-INCH HEELS)		SMALL FRAME	MEDIUM FRAME	LARGE FRAME
Feet	Inches			
5	2	112-120	118-129	126-141
5	3	115-123	121-133	129-144
5	4	118-126	124-136	132-148
5	5	121-129	127-139	135-152
5	6	124-133	130-143	138-156
5	7	128-137	134-147	142-161
5	8	132-141	138-152	147-166
5	9	136-145	142-156	151-170
5	10	140-150	146-160	155-174
5	11	144-154	150-165	159-179
6	0	148-158	154-170	164-184
6	1	152-162	158-175	168-189
6	2	156-167	162-180	173-194
6	3	160-171	167-185	178-199
6	4	164-175	172-190	182-204

SOURCE: Metropolitan Life Insurance Company.

Desirable Weights for Women of Ages 25 and Over: Weight in Pounds According to Frame (in Indoor Clothing)[a]

HEIGHT (WITH SHOES ON— 2-INCH HEELS)		SMALL FRAME	MEDIUM FRAME	LARGE FRAME
Feet	*Inches*			
4	10	92- 98	96-107	104-119
4	11	94-101	98-110	106-122
5	0	96-104	101-113	109-125
5	1	99-107	104-116	112-128
5	2	102-110	107-119	115-131
5	3	105-113	110-122	118-134
5	4	108-116	113-126	121-138
5	5	111-119	116-130	125-142
5	6	114-123	120-135	129-146
5	7	118-127	124-139	133-150
5	8	122-131	128-143	137-154
5	9	126-135	132-147	141-158
5	10	130-140	136-151	145-163
5	11	134-144	140-155	149-168
6	0	138-148	144-159	153-173

[a]For girls between 18 and 25, subtract 1 pound for each year under 25.

SOURCE: Metropolitan Life Insurance Company.

GLOSSARY

Abduction: Movement of part of the body away from the midline of the body.

Adduction: Movement of part of the body toward the midline of the body.

Agility: Ability to change direction quickly and effectively while moving as nearly as possible at full speed.

Appestat: A popularized name for the centers in the hypothalamus that regulate appetite and satiety.

Atherosclerosis: Fatty degeneration and deposits in and on the inner wall of an artery.

Balance: Ability to maintain one's equilibrium while stationary and while moving in various ways at various speeds.

Blood Platelets: Small blood cells necessary for blood clotting.

Body Density: The relative weight of the body compared with an equal volume of water.

Calorie: The heat required to raise the temperature of one kilogram of water from 14.5°C. to 15.5°C.

Carbohydrate: A major energy-yielding organic compound found in sugars, starches, and cellulose.

Cardiac Output: Volume of blood pumped by the heart in 1 minute; at rest, about 5 liters per minute in an average-sized man.

Center of Gravity: The theoretical point in a body (or body part) where the entire weight of the body can be considered to be acting.

Cholesterol: A waxy organic alcohol classed as a lipid because it acts like a fat, present in animal fats; it is an important building tissue but may be associated with atherosclerosis and coronary heart disease when it appears to excess in the circulating blood.

Circulo-respiratory Fitness (CR Capacity): The quality that enables one to endure in reasonably vigorous physical activity for extended periods of time.

Conditioning: General physiological improvement of the systems of the body.

Coordination: The smooth flow of movement in the execution of a motor task.

Coronary Heart Disease: Narrowing of the coronary arteries (the blood vessels feeding the heart muscle itself).

Dehydration: Loss of body water.

Dynamometer: A mechanical device for measuring force.

Electrolyte: A solution or substance which, in solution, conducts electricity.

Enzyme: An organic catalyst that aids in many body processes such as digestion and oxidation.

Exercise: Conscious and purposeful physical activity, usually of sufficient intensity to increase to some degree respiratory and circulatory functions.

Extension: Increasing the angle of a joint (as in elbow extension, straightening the elbow).

Flexibility: The functional capacity of a joint to move through a normal range of motion.

Flexion: Decreasing the angle of a joint (as in elbow flexion, bending the elbow).

Gluconeogenesis: The conversion of noncarbohydrate substances (fats, proteins) to glucose.

Glycogenolysis: The breakdown of stored glycogen to glucose, usually for energy purposes.

Hamstrings: Collectively, the powerful muscles on the rear of the upper leg; they cause knee flexion and, when the knee is fixed, aid hip extension.

Health: Mental and physical well-being; soundness of mind and body; fitness of the organs and systems of the body and fitness of the mind.

Heat Stroke: Caused by prolonged exposure to high temperatures or the direct rays of the sun, especially likely when humidity also is relatively high; weakness, dizziness, headache, nausea, hot and dry skin are some of the symptoms; if not reversed, may be fatal or may cause brain damage.

Hemoglobin: The oxygen-carrying component of the red blood cell (also carries some of the carbon dioxide).

Heterogeneous: Unlike; not homogeneous.

Hormones: Chemical products, secreted by the endocrine glands into the blood; each exerts a definite influence on some specific body organ or function.

Hypertrophy: Increase in size of tissue or organ due to enlargement of cells, not due to increased number of cells.

Hypothalamus: The most anterior part of the brain stem called the diencephalon.

Inhibition-facilitation Ratio: A central nervous system phenomenon, which neurologically aids or limits muscle function.

Intensity: Difficulty of effort as opposed to duration of effort (for example, sprinting is more intensive than jogging, lifting 100 pounds is more intensive than lifting 25 pounds).

Isometric Strength: Refers to amount of force one can exert against a fixed resistance during one all-out exertion.

Isotonic Strength: Refers to amount of resistance one can overcome during one application of force through the full range of motion of the particular joint or joints of the body that are involved.

Lactic Acid: An end product of glucose oxidation, which is formed when inadequate oxygen is present to complete oxidation.

Maximal Oxygen Utilization: The maximal amount of oxygen that can be extracted by the tissues per minute.

Metabolism: The sum total of all the body's energy processes, including the storing and use of energy.

Mineral: A natural inorganic element or compound; those required by the body are essential to normal organic processes.

Motor Ability: The ability to carry out a particular motor function.

Motor Capacity: The extent to which one can develop his motor abilities.

Motor Educability: One's ability to adapt to and learn new movements or activities that depend to a high degree on motor performance.

Movement Time: The time period necessary to move a part of the body from one point to another.

Muscular Endurance: The quality that enables one to persist in localized muscle group activities for extended periods of time.

Overload: The great demands that must be placed on a system if significant changes are to occur in physical fitness.

Oxidative Process: The process of chemical change, which involves combination with oxygen; for example, energy is released and CO_2 and H_2O are formed when glucose is oxidized.

Oxygen Debt: The amount of oxygen used *after* exercise that is over and above resting O_2 utilization; the debt or "deficit" builds up during exercise whenever O_2 utilization is less than O_2 requirement.

Oxygen Debt Tolerance: The maximum oxygen debt a person can build up before he ceases exercising.

Oxygen Requirement: The amount of oxygen needed by the body to carry out a given task; may be expressed as a rate (milliliters per minute) or total amount for a task.

Oxygen Utilization: The amount of oxygen actually used by the body per unit of time; usually expressed in liters or milliliters per minute; at rest, averages about 200-300 ml. per min., depending on body size.

Physical Fitness: The capacity to carry out moderate to strenuous physical tasks, especially those that require well-conditioned neuromuscular and circulo-respiratory systems.

Plasma: The liquid or solvent portion of blood.

Power: A great amount of force applied over a short period of time to achieve explosive movement of the body.

Protein: A food compound composed of amino acids; essential to all living organisms for growth and repair of tissues.

Reaction Time: The length of time required to initiate a response to a specific stimulus.

Response Time: Total time elapsed from the stimulus to the completion of the neuromuscular response.

Retrogression: A period of leveling off or even falling off in performance that may occur after some improvement has already taken place.

Rotation: Joint action that involves turning on an axis.

Saturated Fat: Hard fats, saturated with hydrogen atoms. They are apparently associated with atherosclerosis more than are unsaturated fats.

Simple Sugars: Glucose, lactose, and galactose; one-molecule carbohydrates.

Specificity: The principle that the best way to improve one's fitness for a particular activity is to practice that activity itself, or one that simulates as nearly as possible the activity one wishes to improve.

Speed: The movement of the entire body rapidly from one place to another.

Spleen: An organ located near the stomach; it is not well understood, but is known to contain blood especially rich in red blood cells.

Strength: Maximal force exerted one time.

Stroke Volume: Amount of blood pumped by the heart in one contraction; about 70 ml. per beat in a resting man.

Systolic Blood Pressure: The blood pressure attained during the peak of the contraction phase of the cardiac cycle.

Training: A process directed at the improvement of a specific performance.

Unsaturated Fats: "Soft" fats, usually liquid at room temperature; fats not saturated with hydrogen atoms.

Vital Capacity: The maximal expiration possible after a maximal inspiration.

Vitamins: Non-caloric nutrients, each essential to some normal body function.

Weight Lifting: A competitive effort to lift a maximal amount of weight.

White Blood Cells: Blood cells which act as scavengers and aid in resistance to infection.

Work Capacity: The maximal length of time a given work task can be continued.

SELECTED REFERENCES
AND READINGS

Adult physical fitness. 1963. Washington, D.C.: Government Printing Office, No. 0-705-236.

Anderson, Kenneth A. 1961. The effect of the weighted ankle spat on the jumping performance, agility, and endurance of high school basketball players. (Master's thesis, University of Wisconsin) Madison, Wisc.: University Microfilms, No. 96P.

Bachman, J.C., Horvath, S.M. 1968. Pulmonary function changes which accompany athletic conditioning programs. *Research Quarterly* 39:232.

Baker, J.A. 1968. Comparison of rope skipping and jogging as methods of improving cardiovascular efficiency of college men. *Research Quarterly* 39:240.

Balke, B., Clark, R.T. 1961. Cardio-pulmonary and metabolic effects of physical training, in *Health and fitness in the modern world.* Chicago: The Athletic Institute.

Banister, Eric W. 1963. The relative effectiveness of interval circuit training compared with three other methods of fitness training in a high school physical education program. (Unpublished master's thesis, University of British Columbia.)

Berger, R.A. 1962. Comparison of static and dynamic strength increases. *Research Quarterly* 33:329.

Berger, R.A. 1962. Optimum repetitions for the development of strength. *Research Quarterly* 33:334.

Berger, R.A. 1963. Classification of students on the basis of strength. *Research Quarterly* 34:514.

Berger, R.A. 1963. Comparison between static training and various dynamic training programs. *Research Quarterly* 34:131.

Berger, R.A. 1965. Comparison of the effect of various weight training loads on strength. *Research Quarterly* 36:141.

Berger, R.A. 1966. Relationship of chinning strength to dynamic strength. *Research Quarterly* 37:431.

Berger, R.A. 1967. Determination of a method to predict 1-RM chin and dip from repetitive chins and dips. *Research Quarterly* 38:330.

Berger, R.A. 1967. Effect of maximum loads for each of ten repetitions on strength improvement. *Research Quarterly* 38:715.

Berger, R.A., Bluschke, L.A. 1967. Comparison of relationships between motor ability and static and dynamic strength. *Research Quarterly* 38: 144-146.

Bowerman, W.J., Harris, W.E. 1967. *Jogging*. New York: Grosset and Dunlap, 1967.

Brunner, D., Manelis, G. 1960. Myocardial infarction among members of communal settlements in Israel. *Lancet* Nov. 12, p. 1049.

Capen, E.K. 1950. The effect of systematic weight training on power, strength, and endurance. *Research Quarterly* 21:83.

Casady, D.R. et al. 1965. *Handbook of physical fitness activities*. New York: MacMillan.

Chapman, C.B., Mitchell, J.H. 1965. The physiology of exercise. *Scientific American* 212:88.

Chui, E.F. 1964. Effects of isometric and dynamic weight-training exercises upon strength and speed of movement. *Research Quarterly* 35:246.

Clarke, H.H. 1957. *Application of measurement to health and physical education.* Englewood Cliffs, N.J.: Prentice-Hall.

Clarke, H.H., Bailey, T.L., Shay, C.T. 1952. New objective strength tests of muscle groups by cable-tension methods. *Research Quarterly* 23:136.

Cooper, K.H. 1968. *Aerobics*. New York: Bantam.

Cotton, D. 1967. Relationship of the duration of sustained voluntary contraction to changes in endurance and strength. *Research Quarterly* 38:366.

Cowell, C.C. 1960. The contributions of physical activity to social development. *Research Quarterly* 31:286.

Cratty, B.J. 1967. *Social dimensions of physical activity.* Englewood Cliffs, N.J.: Prentice-Hall.

Cureton, T.K. 1951. *Physical fitness of champion athletes.* Urbana, Ill.: University of Illinois Press.

Fabry, P. et al. 1964. The frequency of meals: its relation to overweight, hypercholesterolemia, and decreased glucose-tolerance. *Lancet* Sept. 19, p. 614.

Flint, M.M. 1968. Effect of increasing back and abdominal muscle strength on low back pain. *Research Quarterly* 39:170.

Frank, J.H. 1967. Comparison of pre- and postfitness scores in a conditioning experiment. *Research Quarterly* 38:510.

Green, R.M., trans. 1951. Galen's *De sanitate tuenda*. Springfield, Ill.: Charles C Thomas. Cited by L.E. Morehouse and P.J. Rasch in *Scientific basis of athletic training.* Philadelphia: W.B. Saunders.

Hakes, R.R., Rosemier, R.A. 1967. Circuit training time allotments in a physical education class period. *Research Quarterly* 38:576.

Hammond, E.G. 1964. Some preliminary findings on physical complaints from a prospective study of 1,064,004 men and women. *American Journal of Public Health* 54:11.

The healthy life. 1966. New York: Time Incorporated.

Hedley, O.F. 1939. Analysis of 5116 deaths reported as due to acute coronary occlusion in Philadelphia 1933-1937. United States *Weekly Public Health Reports*. 54:972.

Helixon, P. 1961. The effects of progressive heavy resistance exercises using near-maximum weights on the running and jumping ability of first year high school track performers. University of Wisconsin, unpublished master's thesis.

Henry, F.M. 1954. Influence of athletic training on the resting cardiovascular system. *Research Quarterly* 25:28.

Howell, M.L., Morford, W.R. 1961. Circuit training. *Journal of Health, Physical Education and Recreation 32:33*.

Howell, M.L., Morford, W.R. 1964. Circuit training for a college fitness program. *Journal of Health, Physical Education and Recreation* 35:30.

Johnson, P.B. 1968. Metabolism and weight control. *Journal of Health, Physical Education and Recreation* 39:39.

Johnson, P.B., Cooper, J. 1967. The effects of meal eating, nibbling, and starvation-refeeding in male albino rats. Paper presented at Research Section, AAHPER National Convention, Las Vegas.

Johnson, P.B., Updyke, W.F., Henry, W. 1965. Effect of regular exercise on diurnal variation in submaximal metabolism. *Abstracts of Research Papers*, AAHPER Convention.

Johnson, P.B., Updyke, W.F., Stolberg, D.C., Schaefer, M. 1966. *Physical education: problem-solving approach to health and fitness*. New York: Holt, Rinehart and Winston.

Johnson, W., Kramer, G.F. 1961. Effects of stereotyped non-hypnotic,

hypnotic and post-hypnotic suggestions upon strength, power and endurance. *Research Quarterly* 32:522-529.

Jones, D.M., Squires, C., Rodahl, K. 1962. The effect of rope skipping on physical work capacity. *Research Quarterly* 33:236.

Jones, E.M. et al. 1964. Effects of exercise and food restriction on serum cholesterol and liver lipids. *American Journal of Physiology* 207:460.

Jones, R.E. 1968. A neurological interpretation of isometric exercise. *Research Quarterly* 39:1126.

Karpovich, P.V. 1965. *Physiology of muscular activity*. Philadelphia: W.B. Saunders.

Kenyon, G.S. 1968. Claims for physical exercise and formal physical education: fact and fancy concerning psychological and sociological benefits: sociological considerations. Paper presented at Scientific Foundations Section, AAHPER Convention, St. Louis.

Kjellberg, S.R., Rudhe, V., Sjostrand, T. 1949. Increase in the amount of hemoglobin and blood volume in connection with physical training. *Acta Physiologica Scandinavica* 19:146.

Knehr, C.A., Dill, D.B., Newfeld, W. 1942. Training and its effects on man at rest and at work. *American Journal of Physiology* 136:148.

Kozar, A.J., Hunsicker, P. 1963. A study of telemetered heart rate during sports participations of young adult men. *Journal of Sports Medicine and Physical Fitness* 3:1.

Kraus, N., Raab, W. 1961. *Hypokinetic disease*. Springfield, Ill.: Charles C Thomas.

Kroll, W. 1966. Level of isometric strength and isometric endurance in repeated contractions. *Research Quarterly* 37:375.

Mallerowicz, H. 1960. The effects of training on O_2 consumption of the heart and its importance for prevention of coronary insufficiency, in *Health and Fitness in the Modern World*. Chicago: The Athletic Institute.

Martens, R., Sharkey, B.J. 1966. Relationship of phasic and static strength and endurance. *Research Quarterly* 37:435.

Massey, B.H. et al. 1959. *The kinesiology of weight lifting*. Dubuque, Iowa: Wm. C. Brown.

Mayer, J. 1960. Exercise and weight control. *Science and medicine of exercise and sports*. New York: Harper and Row.

Mayer, J., Bullen, B. 1960. Nutrition and athletic performance, in *Exercise and fitness*. Chicago: The Athletic Institute.

McGavack, T.H. 1965. Optimal weight determination: experiences with the method of Willoughby as a guide to reduction. *Metabolism* 14:150.

Meyers, C.R. 1967. Effects of two isometric routines on strength, size and endurance in exercised and nonexercised arms. *Research Quarterly* 38:430.

Moncrieff, J. 1963. Variations in the effect of two training methods upon work output. Vancouver, B.C.: University Microfilms, No. 58P. Master's thesis, University of British Columbia.

Montoye, J.H. 1960. Sports and length of life, in W.R. Johnson (ed.), *Science and medicine of exercise and sports*. New York: Harper and Row.

Montoye, J.H. et al. 1957. *Longevity and morbidity of college athletes*. Indianapolis: Phi Epsilon Kappa Fraternity.

Morehouse, C.A. 1967. Development and maintenance of isometric strength of subjects with diverse initial strengths. *Research Quarterly* 38:449.

Morehouse, L.E., Miller, A.T. 1963. *Physiology of exercise*. St. Louis, Mo.: C.V. Mosby.

Morgan, R.E., Adamson, C.T. 1959. *Circuit training.* London: G. Bell and Sons.

Morris, J.N., Crawford, M.D. 1958. Coronary heart disease and physical activity of work, evidence of national necropsy study. *British Medical Journal* 2:1485.

Morris, J.N. et al. 1953. Coronary heart disease and physical activity of work. *Lancet* 2:1053.

Murray, J., Karpovich, P.V. 1957. *Weight training in athletics*. Englewood Cliffs, N.J.: Prentice-Hall.

O'Shea, J.P. 1969. Scientific principles and methods of strength and fitness. Reading, Mass.: Addison-Wesley.

Parizkova, J., Stankova, L. 1964. Influence of physical activity on a treadmill on the metabolism of adipose tissue in rats. *British Journal of Nutrition* 18:325.

Pedley, F.G. 1942. Coronary disease and occupation. *Canadian Medical Association Journal* 40:147.

Plato. *The republic*. Trans. B. Jowett. 1928. New York: Modern Library.

Present knowledge of carbohydrates. 1966. *Nutrition Review* 24:65.

Present knowledge of fat. 1966. *Nutrition Review* 24:33.

Radford, E., Radford, M.A. 1949. *Encyclopedia of superstitions*. New York: Philosophical Library.

Rasch, P.J. 1966. *Weight training.* Dubuque, Iowa: Wm. C. Brown.

Ricci, B. 1966. *Physical and physiological conditioning for men.* Dubuque, Iowa: Wm. C. Brown.

Royce, J. 1964. Re-evaluation of isometric training methods and results, a must. *Research Quarterly* 35:215.

Ryle, J.A., Russel, W.T. 1949. The national history of coronary disease. *British Heart Journal* 11:370.

Schwartz, L., Britten, R.H., Thompson, L.R. 1928. Studies in physical development and posture: the effects of exercise on the physical condition and development of adolescent boys. *Public Health Bulletin* 179:1.

Seyffarth, H. 1940. The behavior of motor units in voluntary contraction. *Skr. Worke Vidnsk Akad. I Mat-Nat. Kl.* 4:17.

Sharkey, B., Holleman, J.P. 1967. Cardio-respiratory adaptations to training at specific intensities. *Research Quarterly* 38:698.

Singer, R. N. 1968. *Motor learning and human performance: an application to physical education skills.* New York: Macmillan.

Solley, W. H. 1952. The effects of verbal instruction of speed and accuracy upon the learning of a motor skill. *Research Quarterly* 23:231.

Sorani, R. 1966. *Circuit training.* Dubuque, Iowa: Wm. C. Brown.

Stamler, J., Kjelsberg, M., Hall, Y. 1960. Epidemiological studies in cardiovascular renal disease in Chicago and Illinois. *Journal of Chronic Diseases* 12:440.

Steinhaus, A.H. 1957. *How to keep fit and like it.* Chicago: The Dartnell Corp.

Steinhaus, A.H. 1963. *Toward an understanding of health and physical education.* Dubuque, Iowa: Wm. C. Brown.

Taylor, H.L. 1960. Exercise and metabolism, in *Science and medicine of exercise and sports.* New York: Harper and Row.

Taylor, H.L. 1960. The mortality and morbidity of coronary heart disease of men in sedentary and physically active occupations, in *Exercise and fitness.* Chicago: The Athletic Institute.

Toynbee, A.J. 1946. *A study of history.* London: Oxford University Press.

Van Dalen, D.B., Mitchell, E.D., Bennett, B.L. 1953. *A world history of physical education.* Englewood Cliffs, N.J.: Prentice-Hall.

Wahlund, H. 1948. Determination of the physical working capacity. *Acta Medicus Scandinavica,* 215:195.

Wikander, G., Johnson, P.B. Unpublished data, University of Toledo.

Wilkins, B.M. 1952. The effect of systematic weight training on speed of movement. *Research Quarterly* 23:361.

Willoughby, D.P. 1932. An anthropometric method for arriving at the optimal proportions of the body in the adult individual. *Research Quarterly* 3:48.

Wishnofsky, M. 1958. Caloric equivalent of gained or lost weight. *American Journal of Clinical Nutrition* 6:542.

Yost, C.P. 1967. Total fitness and prevention of accidents. *Journal of Health, Physical Education and Recreation* 38:32.

Yudkin, J. 1964. Patterns and trends in carbohydrate consumption and their relation to disease. *Proceedings of Nutrition Society* 23:149.

Yudkin, J., Morland, J. 1967. Sugar intake and myocardial infarction. *The American Journal of Clinical Nutrition* 20:503.

Zauner, C.W., Burt, J.J., Mapes, D.F. 1968. Effect of strenuous and mild pre-meal exercise on postprandial lipemia. *Research Quarterly* 39:395.

Zauner, C.W., Mapes, D. 1965. The effect of pre-meal exercise on the rate of clearing of postprandial lipemia with the factor of intestinal absorption eliminated. Paper presented at Eastern AAHPER meetings.

Zimkin, N.V. 1961. Stress during muscular exercises and the state of non-specifically increased resistance. *Physiological Journal of the USSR* 47:741.

Zucatto, F., Drowatzky, J.N. 1967. Interrelationships between static and dynamic balance. *Research Quarterly* 38:509.

Zukel, W.J. et al. 1959. A short term community study of the epidemiology of coronary heart disease. *Journal of Public Health* 49:1630.

INDEX